The Management of Medical Emergencies:
A Guide for Dental Care Professionals

The Management of Medical Emergencies:
A Guide for Dental Care Professionals

By

Colette Balmer and Lesley Longman

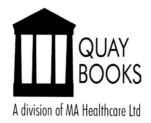

QUAY
BOOKS

A division of MA Healthcare Ltd

Quay Books Division, MA Healthcare Ltd, St Jude's Church, Dulwich Road, London
SE24 0PB

British Library Cataloguing-in-Publication Data
A catalogue record is available for this book

Printed by Ashford Colour Press Ltd, Gosport, Hants,

Contents

Contributors

Dr Colette Balmer
BSc, BChD, FDSRCS(Ed), PCTLCP, FHEA
Consultant in Oral Surgery, Liverpool University Dental Hospital,
and Associate Postgraduate Dental Dean at the Mersey Deanery

Colette gained a BSc(hons) in Microbiology in 1979 and then studied
Dentistry at Leeds Dental School, qualifying in 1983. She gained her FDS in
1987 and followed a career in oral surgery. Colette has always been involved
in the teaching of dental undergraduates, dental postgraduates and dental
care professionals, and has a Postgraduate Teaching Certificate, a Diploma
in Clinical Education, and is a Fellow of the Higher Education Academy.
Since 1990 Colette has been involved with designing and delivering medical
emergency courses and is qualified as an Advanced Life Support instructor
for the Resuscitation Council UK.

Dr Lesley P Longman
BSc, BDS, FDSRCS(Ed), PhD
Consultant in Restorative Dentistry and Honorary Senior Lecturer,
Liverpool University Dental Hospital

Lesley gained a BSc(Hons) in Pharmacology at Liverpool University in 1977
and then studied Dentistry at Liverpool Dental School, qualifying in 1981.
She gained her FDS in 1984 and followed a career in Restorative Dentistry,
initially as an academic. She obtained a PhD in 1991. In 1997 Lesley moved
to the NHS for a Consultancy. She is Clinical and Teaching Lead for Sedation
and Special Care Dentistry and teaches on undergraduate and postgaduate
medical emergencies courses.

Acknowledgements

The authors would like to acknowledge the help of the Department of Resuscitation and Training at University Hospital Aintree for their help in the production of the photographs, and Miss Caroline Foster for acting as our model.

Colette would like to dedicate this book to her mother Maureen Balmer and her late father Norbert Balmer for their unfailing love and support.

Lesley would like to dedicate this book to her husband Peter.

Foreword

Around 300,000 people visit the dentist every day in England. A medical emergency could potentially occur during any of these visits. The sheer numbers mean it is likely that every dental care professional will at some stage in their career be faced with dealing, as part of a team, with a medical emergency. Increasingly, as patients with complex medical problems lead fuller and longer lives, the chance of encountering medical emergencies within the dental practice are even further increased.

Dealing effectively with medical emergencies is of vital importance as it can, and often does, save lives. All members of the dental team need to have comprehensive training in the management of such emergencies, so that, if they are called upon to manage such a situation, they have both the knowledge and the confidence to tackle emergencies appropriately. Competency around management of medical emergencies is a core requirement of continuous professional development and therefore fundamental to maintain registration on the General Dental Council register. Indeed, our patients have a right to expect that all members of the dental team are proficient in the management of such emergencies.

I spent over 25 years in a general dental practice and we dealt with a range of medical emergencies over that time. They ranged from simple fainting in the waiting room, through epileptic fits and hypoglycaemia, to a cardiac arrest following general anaesthesia in the primary care setting. This last example should certainly now not occur, but other emergencies will continue to occur. As the role of dental care professionals increasingly expands within primary care dental services, providing more complex treatments and increasingly, possibly, working without a dentist on site, it is imperative that this group of professionals have the necessary preparation to be able to handle medical emergencies in the most effective and timely manner.

Dealing with any medical emergency is extremely stressful, and the importance of good quality and regular training, along with hands on simulated role play, cannot be underestimated.

I was delighted to be asked to write the foreword for this book. I am certain it will prove to be a valuable resource in assisting the primary care dental team both in training around this vitally important subject, as well as updating and maintaining the competencies around dealing with medical emergencies in clinical dental practice. It is to be hoped that it will be used by all members of the team to enable them to both train together and work together to improve outcomes for patients.

Dr Barry Cockcroft, Chief Dental Officer

Introduction

A wide range of people visit a dental surgery during the course of an ordinary working day. Examples include practice staff, regular, new and prospective patients (often accompanied by relatives and friends) dental company representatives, potential job applicants and service personnel. The health of these visitors will be variable and sometimes unknown. It is not surprising therefore that any of these individuals may become unwell and need urgent treatment. As healthcare professionals all members of staff should have the ability to provide immediate care for medical emergencies that may arise in a dental surgery setting.

What is a Medical Emergency?

A medical emergency can be described as any situation in which a patient becomes ill. They may or may not lose consciousness, but ultimately their life may be at risk due to a failure of an effective oxygenated circulation to the brain and vital organs.

In order to remain alive all human beings have several essential basic requirements. Fundamentally there must be:

- An adequate supply of oxygen available for gas exchange to be possible in the alveoli of the lungs. This means that air needs to be able to flow into the upper airway in order that oxygen can enter the alveoli (or air sacks) of the lungs. The lower airway consisting of the trachea, bronchi and alveoli must be clear of obstruction and patent to allow the passage of oxygen and gases both in and out of the lungs.
- Sufficient blood supply being pumped around the body to the important organs — the lungs, the brain and the heart. In other words the cardiovascular system needs to be working to ensure that vital organs receive the oxygen they need to continue to function.
- A functioning brain and the nervous system that is in overall control.

A medical emergency will arise when there is a failure in one or more of these pivotal core systems, and unless function can be restored or compensated for it will quickly progress to a shutdown of the other essential organs. The basic functions of the respiratory, cardiovascular and nervous systems are described later in separate chapters. Knowledge of these organ systems and how they depend on each other — their interrelationships — is helpful in understanding what goes wrong when a patient becomes acutely ill and why certain procedures are followed during a medical emergency. It allows you to decide what actions are required urgently and what procedures can be delayed for a short time.

When assisting in, or managing, a medical emergency in a dental environment it is important to remember that the team do not always have to identify the cause of the problem or make an accurate diagnosis. Many of the initial presentations of the various emergencies that may occur can be very similar. It may take time, expertise and special investigations for the underlying causes and sequence of events to be identified. The aim of the dental team is to take care of the patient until specialist help arrives and the patient can be safely transferred to a hospital. The team are undertaking a holding operation. The management of the emergency is, however, dependent upon a systematic assessment of the patient to identify which of the fundamental elements is impaired or missing and providing effective compensation for this. *Table 1* below identifies the primary problem in some medical emergencies. This is a simplistic view, but can be helpful is understanding and managing an emergency.

Prevention of Medical Emergencies

Although it is impossible to prevent the occurrence of all medical emergencies there are many steps that can be taken to reduce the likelihood of such an

---

Table 1   **Medical emergencies and the usual primary system affected**

Faints	Cardiovascular
Fits/seizures	Nervous
Anaphylaxis	Cardiovascular
Hypoglycaemia	Nervous
Asthma	Respiratory: lower airway
Choking	Respiratory: upper airway
Angina	Cardiovascular
Myocardial infarction	Cardiovascular
Stroke	Nervous
Respiratory arrest	Respiratory
Cardiac arrest	Cardiovascular
Panic attack (hyperventilation)	Respiratory

event happening. This starts with identifying those patients who might be expected to have an increased risk of experiencing an adverse medical event. In essence you undertake a risk assessment for each patient. All patients who attend for dental treatment should have been questioned about their past and current medical history, and details of any current medications they may be taking. When there is confusion or doubt around a person's medical history then clarification from the patient's general medical practitioner should be sought before starting any treatment. It is always advisable to confirm that patients have taken their medications as normal on the day of attendance. When a patient uses *rescue* medication for a chronic condition, such as an inhaler for asthma, or GTN spray for angina, it is good practice to check that the patient has this with them and where it is located. If they have not brought their *rescue* medication then it is prudent to have the equivalent medication from the surgery's emergency supplies easily to hand. It is also best practice to confirm the circumstances in which the patient may use this drug and the dose they normally take — this should be documented for reference.

Patients with serious and debilitating conditions need extra consideration and may require extra care and attention. Acknowledging this requirement has the additional benefit of reassuring both the patient and the dental team. Careful and thorough questioning is necessary to help the dental treatment go smoothly and maximise patient care. An example of the type of questions to ask can be illustrated with patients who have chronic breathing problems such as emphysema or bronchitis (also known as chronic obstructive pulmonary disease — COPD). Ask the patient if they become breathless when lying flat; attention is required to the position of the dental chair. Some patients with lung disease may panic if they feel that they cannot breathe and may tolerate poorly a mouthful of water from the air turbine. Efficient aspiration of water and debris is therefore required to prevent the patient becoming distressed or anxious.

Some illnesses impair a patient's mobility or ability to handle stress. A patient with limited function of their limbs may be dependent upon a carer. Consideration should therefore be given to appointment times that are influenced by carers' schedules and availability of transport. Many patients are anxious about receiving dental care and many will not openly admit to their anxieties. All dental care professionals should be aware of the possibility of patients having dental anxiety and try to reduce their stress levels. It is particularly important to minimise anxiety in patients who have medical conditions that can be exacerbated by stress; examples include angina, hypertension, asthma and epilepsy. When patients suffer from chronic conditions it is always helpful to ask the person how they are feeling that day, if it is a good day with respect to their health or are they feeling unwell. It in not wise to undertake elective dental treatment if a patient is feeling ill.

In addition, anyone with chronic disease may tire easily and may not be amenable to long appointments. *Table 2* gives examples of conditions that may have an effect on the provision of dental treatment, more details of some specific conditions are included in other sections of the book.

Table 2   Conditions that may influence the dental management of a patient

Condition	Consider
Insulin dependent diabetes	• Timing of appointments should avoid interference with meal times
Renal Dialysis	• Timing of appointments as patients may be tired after dialysis and may prefer treatments on days when dialysis is not taking place
Chronic respiratory problems	• Chair position may be important • Appointments may need to be of short duration • Have rescue medication readily available • Efficient aspiration
Cardiac problems	• Chair position may be important • Appointments may need to be of short duration • Reduce stress • Have rescue medication readily available
Anticoagulant medication	• Ask patient what their ideal INR range is meant to be and ask if it has been stable • INR value should be known before extraction and surgery • Why is the patient on warfarin?
Allergies	• A full history essential to ensure that allergens are avoided. Type I allergies to latex and penicillins are examples that may influence dental management

Continued...

Epilepsy	• Need to know if there are any provoking stimuli, if there is a pre-seizure aura phase, how well controlled are the seizures, when was the last seizure, what form do the seizures take and how long to they last including the best way to allow recovery to take place
Pregnancy	• Chair position, in the late stages of pregnancy, may be important • Timing of appointments — take into consideration morning sickness • Certain prescribed drugs may not be suitable for use

Preparation of the Dental Team

All staff should be familiar with the location of the emergency equipment and drugs kits in the practice. The current recommended emergency equipment is given in *Table 3*. Guidance on equipment and emergency drugs does change and therefore it is imperative that staff regularly check that the surgery is still compliant with current regulations. All drugs and equipment must be checked regularly to ensure that the drugs are still in date and the equipment is in working order.

Regular in-house practice should be held for the whole dental team, with team members taking it in turns to 'manage' the emergency. Non-clinical staff have a vital role to play and it is essential that they understand the importance of the various tasks members of the team undertake. Staff must be able to carry out effective basic life support (BLS), and this must be certificated and updated annually. Ideally rehearsal of BLS should occur in the practice environment on a regular basis and more frequently than once a year. It is prudent not only to train as a team in BLS, but also in the management of the common medical emergencies that may be encountered. Each individual skill that may be required should be practised so that each team member gains competence and confidence in all aspects of management. This is essential to avoid the confusion and panic that can arise in teams who do not rehearse. This training can easily be incorporated into a BLS training session, and should finish with a 'team debrief' to explore what went particularly well, and which areas might be improved upon. Some dental teams have a clear role or responsibility assigned to individuals; for example one person's job is to get the drugs and

Table 3   Emergency equipment

Pocket mask with one-way valve and oxygen inlet[1]
Self-inflating bag, valve and mask with reservoir in various sizes
Oropharyngeal airways[2] (various sizes)
Nasopharyngeal airways (various sizes)
Oxygen therapy masks with tubing and appropriate connectors for oxygen cylinder
Syringes and needles to deliver emergency drugs by IM and SC routes
IV cannulae and adhesive tape[3]
Independently powered portable suction apparatus with wide bore aspiration tips
Blood pressure monitor[4]
Pulse oximeter[4]
Automated external defibrillator[5]

[1] Equipment should be free from rubber latex and resuscitation equipment must be available in suitable sizes for children

[2] These are also referred to a Gueldel's airway

[3] Only essential in a practice that does IV sedation

[4] Essential in a practice that does IV sedation but valuable when assessing an unwell patient

equipment and draw up any required drugs, another person's role is to ring for the paramedics and note down the time and sequence of events, etc. Whilst this is a very structured and organised approach consideration has to be given to multitasking, as staff may be on annual or sick leave.

There are local courses available on both basic and immediate life support (ILS).

SECTION 1

Fundamental Systems
of the Body

CHAPTER I

Fundamentals of the Respiratory System

An effective functioning respiratory system is the first essential step in delivering oxygen to the organs and tissues of the body. In the assessment of a medical emergency it is always necessary to check the patency of the airway and this should be evaluated at a very early stage of the assessment; ideally it should be the first system the healthcare professional evaluates. This is in accordance with the ABCDE approach to managing medical emergencies as advocated by the Resuscitation Council (UK). The following chapters of this book will use the ABCDE protocol and this system is described in Chapter 7.

The airway is divided into two sections, the 'upper' airway which is above the larynx and consists of the mouth and nose, and the 'lower' airway which consists of the trachea, bronchial tree and the lung alveoli. When we are in a room full of people it is very unusual to be able to hear anyone breathing — if you can it is often indicative of a form of airway obstruction. The type of noise that can be heard and when it occurs (eg. on breathing in or breathing out) is diagnostic of the location of the obstruction.

KEY POINTS

- **A silent airway is either completely open and patent, or totally blocked.**

- **A noisy airway indicates partial obstruction.**

Upper Airway Obstruction

This produces a noise on *inspiration* and may be caused by foreign bodies blocking the laryngeal inlet such as food, pieces of tooth or restorations dislodged during dental treatment, or fluids collecting in the back of the oropharynx such as saliva, water or vomit. Irritation to the larynx and oropharynx can produce swelling and vocal chord spasm. In addition, the tongue can fall backwards to contact the soft palate and produce occlusion of the upper airway. *Table 1.1* lists the noise produced by different types of obstructions.

Table 1.1   Upper airway noises

Noise	Cause
Gurgling	Fluid
Snoring	Tongue obstruction
Crowing	Laryngeal spasm
Stridor	Foreign body

Upper Airway Management

The Conscious Adult Patient

In a conscious patient the presence of a blockage in the upper airway will result in choking, the patient will typically be very distressed, point to their neck and they will begin to cough very forcibly in an attempt to expel the obstruction. They need to be sitting or standing upright and leaning forwards slightly to produce an effective cough. The patient should be encouraged to cough, and if it is proving ineffective then five back blows should be administered. Back blows are done by asking the patient to lean forward, steadying them with one hand on their chest and administering a short blow to their back between the shoulder blades. If the first blow dislodges the obstruction it is not essential to deliver the rest.

If five back blows prove to be ineffective then the next alternative is to administer abdominal thrusts. These can be difficult to do, particularly when there is a height discrepancy between the victim and the rescuer. It is also advisable for the victim to attend the local A&E department if this procedure has been carried out as there is a small risk of rupturing the spleen. It is worth remembering that not clearing the obstruction will result in a far worse prognosis than splenic rupture. Abdominal thrusts are carried out with the rescuer standing behind the patient, encircling the abdomen with their arms and placing one fist into the epigastric area, the other hand is used to 'jerk' the fist upwards in an attempt to force residual air upwards through the airway to dislodge the blockage. Abdominal thrusts are shown in *Figure 1.1*. This manoeuvre can be repeated up to five times.

If all such rescue manoeuvres prove ineffective the patient will tire quickly and eventually lose consciousness; at this point cardiopulmonary resuscitation (CPR) must be started immediately. The algorithm for choking is shown below in *Figure 1.2*.

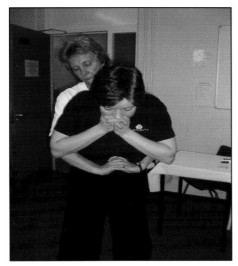

Figure 1.1 Abdominal thrust

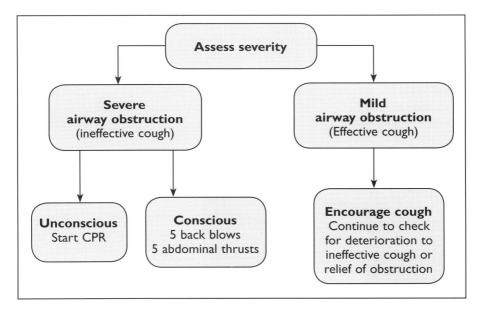

Figure 1.2 Choking algorithm - adult choking treatment.
Source: Reproduced with permission from the Resuscitation Council UK

The Paediatric Patient

A child will become hypoxic very quickly, so effective action to deal with the obstruction is vitally important. There are several differences in the management of a choking child, as opposed to a choking adult, and these are mainly due to the size of the patient and the position of the internal organs. One aspect of the treatment of children that is helpful is the fact that their small size allows the rescuer to use gravitational forces to help dislodge the obstruction as well as the other techniques.

A finger sweep technique should never be used to clear an airway in a child as it is likely to push the obstruction further down the airway, and in addition children tend to have enlarged tonsils and these can be traumatised during a finger sweep, which will result in severe haemorrhage and make the situation worse.

If possible encourage the child to lie prone with the head lower than the feet and administer back blows. If these prove ineffective then abdominal thrusts can be attempted.

If the patient becomes unconscious then administer two effective rescue breathes out of a maximum of five attempts and start CPR immediately.

Babies and infants

These patients should be placed face down over your knee or arm, ensuring that the head of the patient is lower than the feet as shown in *Figure 1.3*.

An alternative is to actually hold them upside down as long as care is taken to support the cervical spine. Five back blows are then administered, remembering to monitor if the obstruction has been dislodged before administering the next blow. If the obstruction remains then the next procedure to try is a 'chest thrust' — where the patient is placed on their back with the head positioned lower than the feet, and five short compressions are

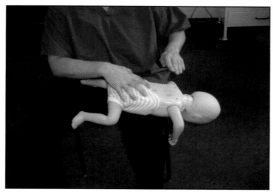

Figure 1.3 Clearing the airway in a choking infant.

applied to the chest in a similar manner to the technique employed during basic life support but using a sharper movement.

Abdominal thrusts should not be carried out on children under one year of age as significant internal organ damage can be caused (see *Figure 1.4*).

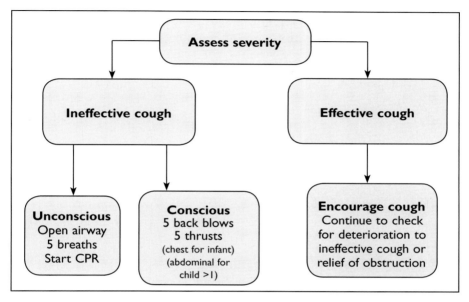

Figure 1.4. Choking algorithm - paediatric choking treatment.
Source: Reproduced with permission from the Resuscitation Council UK

The Unconscious Patient

A patient who is unconscious will require an immediate airway assessment. This is traditionally described as the 'look, listen and feel' approach:

1. **Look** down the line of the patient's chest and observe if there is any movement
2. **Listen** for breath sounds by positioning your ear over the patients mouth and nose, and identify any abnormal sounds as described in *Table 1.1*
3. **Feel** for expired air against your face.

The treatment for an obstructed airway in an unconscious patient depends on the cause of the obstruction. If it is caused by liquids or semi-solid material or foreign bodies in the airway then the position of the patient should be altered to allow gravitational drainage to help. An ideal position is lying the patient over on their side with the head much lower than the feet. Although suction can be helpful it is only really useful for liquids as solid material often occludes the end of the suction apparatus and renders it useless. In addition, suction has to be used with care as inappropriate use can force the obstruction further down the throat.

A finger sweep can be helpful to remove larger objects and semi-solids. A common cause of upper airway obstruction in unconscious patients is the tongue, as shown in *Figure 1.5* below, the tongue relaxes backwards and occludes the airway by lying against the soft palate.

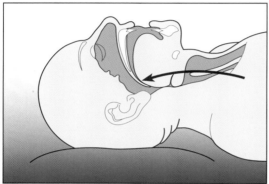

Figure 1.5 Obstruction of the upper airway of the tongue. Source: Resuscitation Council

As the tongue is directly attached to the anterior region of the mandible, by moving the mandible forwards and holding it in this position, the tongue will also move forwards thus re-opening the airway. This is described as a 'jaw thrust' and is carried out by positioning the hands as shown in *Figure 1.6*, and then applying pressure to lift the mandible forwards.

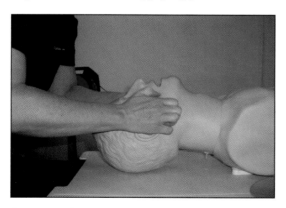

Figure 1.6 A jaw thrust to open the upper airway.

This can be very tiring and difficult to maintain for a long period of time, so an alternative method of opening the airway is usually advocated, this is described as a **head tilt and chin lift,** as illustrated in *Figure 1.7.* The head is elevated off the floor slightly (so as not to produce scrapes on the occiput) and then tilted so the mandible becomes elevated and the tongue moves away from the soft palate. This is not recommended in any patients who may have had cervical spine damage — but this is usually a result of trauma and highly unlikely to occur in a dental surgery setting.

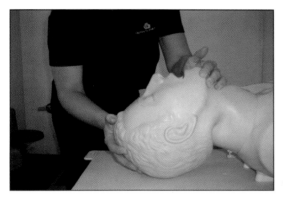

Figure 1.7 Head tilt and chin lift manoeuvre.

Opening the airway in children

Children over one year of age should have the same head position as adults i.e. 'head tilt/ chin lift', but in children under one year of age the head should be kept in a 'neutral' position, i.e. in line with the neck with no tilting or lifting of the chin. This is illustrated in *Figure 1.8* below:

INCORRECT   *CORRECT*

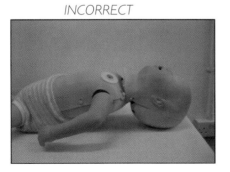
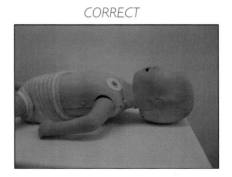

Figure 1.8 Illustrating the correct 'neutral' position when opening the airway in children.

Airway Maintenance Using Simple Adjuncts

In an unconscious patient it may be necessary to maintain the airway using simple adjuncts. These should only be used by staff who have practised the insertion techniques.

Oropharyngeal airway

Oropharyngeal airways (shown in *Figure 1.9*) are designed to control backward displacement of the tongue in the unconscious patient, but head tilt and chin lift will usually need to be maintained.

These airways come in a range of sizes, from newborn to large adult. They are curved rigid tubes, and are flanged and reinforced at the oral end. In adults the most common sizes are 2, 3 and 4 for small, medium and large adult respectively. The correct size of airway requied forn an individual patient is estimated by holding the airway against the jaw so that the flanged end is level with the incisor teeth and the curved end reaches the angle of mandible. This is shown in *Figure 1.10.*

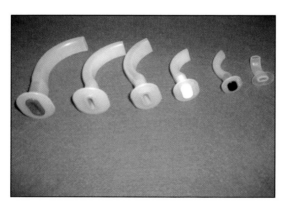

Figure 1.9 Oropharyngeal airways.

CORRECT   TOO LARGE   TOO SMALL

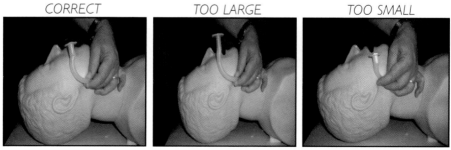

Figure 1.10 Correct sizing for oropharyngeal airways.

They are inserted in to the mouth in the inverted position and rotated through 180 degrees whilst passing under the palate and into the oropharynx, as shown in *Figure 1.11a and 1.11b*. If the patient is only lightly stuporous and laryngeal reflexes are present vomiting, retching, aspiration or laryngospasm may occur. If the patient shows signs of any of the above, remove the airway immediately.

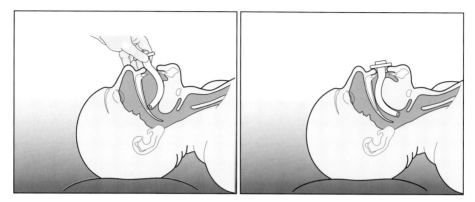

Figures 1.11a and 1.11b Insertion of an oropharyngeal airway.
Adapted from the Resuscitation Council

The nasopharyngeal airway

The nasopharyngeal airway is made from soft plastic, and is far less rigid than the Guedel airway. This airway is flanged at one end and bevelled at the other (*Figure 1.12*).

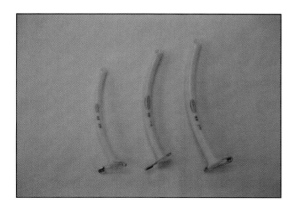

Figure 1.12 Nasopharyngeal airways.

These can be introduced through either nostril, although the right nostril is traditionally used first. The tube will pass through the nasopharynx so the tip is just above the laryngeal opening. Nasopharyngeal airways can be extremely useful in patients with clenched jaws and maxillo-facial injuries. They may also be valuable when the oropharyngeal airway is rejected as they appear to be better tolerated in patients who are not deeply comatose. It must be remembered that these airways must not be used in patients with a suspected basal skull fracture although, again, this scenario is unlikely to be encountered in the dental surgery.

The adult nasopharyngeal sizes are usually 6 to 8mm internal diameter; a quick but effective way of sizing the airway is to compare the tube diameter to that of the patient's little finger.

Having selected the appropriate size, insertion technique is as follows (*Figures 1.13a and 1.13b*):

- Check nostril is patent
- Ensure tube is well lubricated with water soluble lubrication gel, e.g. KY jelly
- Insert safety pin through flange to prevent inhalation of adjunct
- Insert bevel end first, vertically, and twist gently
- When in place, the tip should lie behind the tongue
- If obstruction is met at any stage, withdraw and use other nostril
- Do remember to check patency post-insertion.

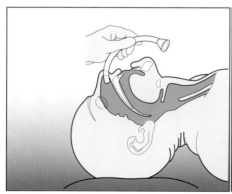 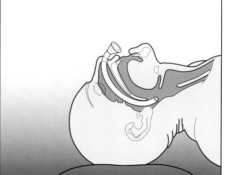

Figure 1.13a Insertion technique.
Adapted from the Resuscitation Council UK

Figure 1.13b Final position of nasopharyngeal airway.
Adapted from the Resuscitation Council UK

Supplemental Oxygen

KEY POINT

Oxygen should be administered in every medical emergency.

If spontaneous respiration is still taking place supplemental oxygen should be administered through an oxygen therapy mask attached to an oxygen supply. A minimum rate of 4-6 litres per minute should be used.

Lower Airway Obstruction

Obstruction of the lower airway produces a noise on **expiration** and is either caused by constriction of the supporting structures, or the presence of excess fluids and secretions in the alveoli and bronchial tree. The diagnosis and management of lower airway obstruction is beyond the scope of this book, but there are two emergency conditions of relevance to the dental surgery; asthma and anaphylaxis. In asthma there is a marked constriction of the bronchi which produces resistance to air movement, and in anaphylaxis the lung tissue begins to fill with fluid and the airways constrict also resulting in increased resistance to air flow. Both conditions result in a marked expiratory wheeze that becomes louder and the respiratory effort becomes more profound as the condition deteriorates. The treatment for both of these conditions is described in detail in the chapters dedicated to anaphylaxis and asthma (Chapters 8 and 10).

Management of lower airway obstruction

Lower airway obstruction cannot be effectively managed in a dental surgery and an ambulance should be called. Supportive therapy with high flow oxygen 10-15 litres per minute should be administered via a suitable delivery system, e.g. a non-rebreatheable mast attached to a cylinder.

Respiratory Arrest

Artificial ventilation is required in patients who have no spontaneous respiration and when the respiration rate is less than 8 breaths per minute.

It is possible to administer expired air respiration — mouth-to-mouth resuscitation. This is difficult to do effectively, may be unaesthetic and only delivers 16% oxygen to the lungs; room air contains 21% oxygen. There are two main adjuncts available to assist in artificial ventilations, which make the procedure acceptable to the operator and also more efficacious. The pocket mask (*Figure 1.14*) and the bag, valve, mask (*Figures 1.15a and b*) are both capable of being connected to supplemental oxygen and whenever there is an oxygen supply available should always be given to the casualty. With both of these adjuncts it is essential to ensure that the upper airway is opened (ie a 'head tilt' and 'chin lift') and maintained throughout.

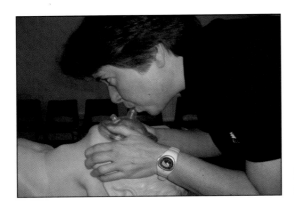

Figure 1.14 Ventilation using the pocket mask.

The main difficulty with the pocket mask is the maintenance of an airtight seal. If the personnel are available it is recommended that one maintains the seal while the other delivers rescue breaths. The mask is usually placed on the patient's face using the thumb and forefingers of both hands, lifting the angles of the jaw with the other fingers to obtain an airtight fit. Blow into the port of the mask to inflate the patients lungs and watch for the chest to rise. Following each rescue breath watch the chest fall to ensure expiration has taken place. If any leaks are noted, adjust hand position and/or contact pressure.

It should be noted that a tidal volume of no greater than 400-500ml/breath should be used in rescue breathing. Over-vigorous breaths can result in gastric insufflation, increasing the risk of regurgitation and pulmonary aspiration. In addition, over-enthusiastic rescue breathing may also lead to high inflation pressures.

Bag-mask

The self-inflating bag with one-way valve is the most common device used on patients with absent spontaneous respiration. The mask is positioned over the patient's mouth in the exact same way as the pocket mask, ensuring an airtight seal. The bag is then squeezed gently to administer a tidal volume of 500ml into the patient's lungs. The lungs are allowed to deflate spontaneously and a further 'breath' is delivered. By connecting the reservoir bag to high flow oxygen the patient could receive 90 % oxygen per ventilation, provided that an effective seal around the mask is produced. It can be difficult to achieve an airtight seal and it is much easier to use a 'two handed' technique, where one rescuer holds the mask in place and the second provides the ventilations.

Paramedics may use other more advanced airway techniques such as insertion of laryngeal mask airways and endotracheal airways, but this equipment is not kept in dental surgeries and dental personnel are not routinely trained in their use.

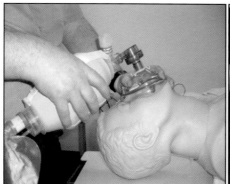 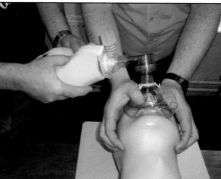

Figure 1.15a Bag-mask: one person technique.

Figure 1.15b Bag-mask: two person technique.

CHAPTER 2

Fundamentals of the Cardiovascular System

In resuscitation terms the cardiovascular system (CVS) can be considered as the body's transport and distribution network for oxygen. There are three main components to the system:

- Blood vessels or circulatory system which distribute substances around the body
- Blood which is the transport medium
- Heart which is effectively a pump to circulate blood throughout the vascular system.

In order to ensure sufficient oxygen is reaching the tissues, particularly the brain, there must be an adequate and continuous blood flow to supply it, which in turn means the system has to be maintained with sufficient pressure to provide this blood flow. The information in this chapter will help the reader understand how a circulation is achieved and what goes wrong in medical emergencies that are primarily caused by a malfunction of the CVS.

Blood Pressure

What is 'blood pressure'?

The heart is essentially comprised of two separate pumps, the right side and the left side. The right side of the heart pumps deoxygenated blood (blood without oxygen) to the lungs, where it collects oxygen and then returns to the left side of the heart. The left side of the heart, specifically the left ventricle, contracts and pumps the oxygenated blood into the aorta. The amount of blood the left ventricle produces at each contraction is called the cardiac output. Each contraction (systole) forces approximately 70ml of blood into the circulation, there is then a pause whilst the ventricle refills (diastole) and then it contracts again ejecting another 70 mls of blood. The sequence of events between one heartbeat and the next is called the cardiac cycle, and this takes around 0.8 seconds to complete. The sequence represents a cycle of work for the heart that comprises of diastole and systole. To summarise, a cardiac cycle consists of the atria contracting together to force the blood into the ventricles. The ventricles then contract simultaneously and pump blood out through the pulmonary artery and aorta. As the ventricles contract the atria are relaxed and fill up again with blood to allow the process to be repeated.

The flow of blood out of the heart is pulsatile, but the supply of oxygenated blood to the tissues and organs needs to be continuous; the elastic recoil of the arteries and arterioles helps to achieve this. Arteries and arterioles have flexibility within the structure of their walls which allows them to expand to accommodate the sudden influx of blood and to return to their resting diameter. The large arteries are quite rigid to resist the power of the pumping action of the left ventricle, but the smaller arteries and particularly the arterioles are more flexible and thus the pulsatile flow is converted into a continuous flow.

The 'pump power' of the left ventricle and the elasticity of the arterial system are the most important factors in measuring blood pressure (BP). When a person's BP is recorded the highest (top) reading — systolic blood pressure — is a measure of the power of the left ventricular contraction. The lower, or diastolic pressure is a measure of the vascular resistance. Blood pressure is measured in 'millimetres of mecury pressure' (mmHg) and a normal systolic blood pressure is quoted as being 120mmHg but this does increase with age: a maximum healthy systolic blood pressure could be broadly defined as 100mmHg plus the patient's age in years. For example, a 60-year-old would be 160mmHg, anything significantly over this is potentially unhealthy and possibly dangerous. A normal diastolic pressure would be around 70–80mmHg, and if it is more than 100mmHg the person is considered to be hypertensive and would require medical assessment.

In resuscitation terms a systolic blood pressure of 90mmHg or below, and a diastolic of 60mmHg or below, is considered to be a very adverse sign and immediate treatment is required. If blood pressure falls there will be insufficient oxygenated blood reaching the brain and the person will become disorientated and eventually unconscious.

What can alter blood pressure?

The systolic and diastolic pressures are interlinked in the sense that if the diastolic pressure goes up the heart has to work harder to push the blood through the vessels, so the systolic pressure will also rise. If the vascular resistance falls the heart does not have to pump as hard and the systolic pressure will drop slightly. The resistance of the vessels is altered either by dilating them — which reduces resistance to blood flow — or by constricting them — which increases the resistance. The force of contraction of the left ventricle is directly influenced by the amount of blood entering it. When more blood enters the left ventricle, more blood needs to be ejected so a more forceful or powerful ventricular contraction is required; this is known as Starling's law of the heart. There are three ways to compensate, therefore, for a fall in blood pressure:

- Increase the peripheral vascular resistance. This can only be done using drugs and would not be possible in a dental surgery setting
- Increase the amount of fluid in the circulatory system. This would automatically increase the amount of blood entering the left ventricle and thus increase the pump power. This requires administration of intravenous fluids and again is not appropriate in a dental surgery
- Increase the amount of blood returning to the heart by redistributing the blood volume. Restoration of the circulatory volume is feasible and appropriate when blood is pooling in the limbs. Laying the patient flat and elevating the legs will very quickly restore an adequate circulatory volume in this situation.

The important point to remember is that altering the position of the dental chair by lying a patient flat will increase the amount of blood returning to the heart and thus increase the power of contraction of the left ventricle. This is an ideal outcome in the case of a simple faint or anaphylaxis but is not ideal in other emergency situations, such as an angina attack. In angina the heart is already struggling to cope, and to force it to work harder is counterproductive. Therefore, unless a person is unconscious, you need to think carefully before lying them flat.

KEY POINT

Altering the position of the dental chair, by lying the patient flat, will increase the amount of blood returning to the heart and thus increase the cardiac output.

Circulation

A 70kg person will have a total blood volume of approximately 5 litres; at any one time approximately 1 litre will be in the lungs, 3 litres in the systemic veins, and the remaining 1 litre will be in the heart, arteries and arterioles, and capillaries. The nervous system can control the diameter of some of the arterioles supplying the periphery of the body. When required, it can redirect the blood flow from the limbs, bowels and skin to increase the supply to the central circulation, which supplies the core organs such as the heart and brain.

An obvious example would be a sudden traumatic injury resulting in a major blood loss, say 1 litre. The blood pressure would fall as a result of the drop in circulating volume, the peripheral circulation would then close down to allow the remaining blood to stay in the central circulation to continue to supply vital organs. This phenomenon is known as 'peripheral venous shutdown' and is a common occurrence in medical emergencies. This is why the patient will appear pale and cold because there is very little blood at the skin surface. The second physical effect of this is that there is very little blood going through the arteries supplying the limbs so the pulses at the wrist will be barely detectable. There will thus be a discrepancy between the qualities of a peripheral and central pulse.

The Heart

The mechanical contraction of the heart is the effect of a wave of depolarisation spreading through the cardiac muscle. This can be considered an electrical impulse which travels through the muscle in a predetermined or predictable manner (see *Figure 2.1*).

The initial wave of depolarisation usually starts in the sinoatrial node (the natural pacemaker) and travels through the atria producing a co-ordinated contraction of the atrial muscle which forces the blood through into the ventricles. There is a small delay as the wave crosses the gap to the atrioventricular node and then it travels down specialised conducting tissue (bundle of His) to the base of the ventricles and up the sides, resulting in co-ordinated ventricular contraction. Once the depolarisation wave has been started it will continue in this predetermined way. A good analogy is a line of dominoes standing on their edges, if you flick the first one it results in a wave of dominoes all falling down. Obviously you could actually tip one of the dominoes in the middle of the line, and all the ones after it will fall over as usual. The same is true of the depolarisation wave, it can be initiated from anywhere within the conduction

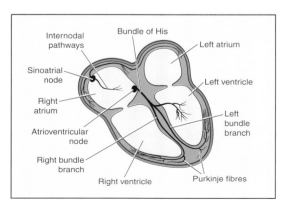

Figure 2.1 The normal cardiac conduction pathway.

system but will only travel in one predetermined direction. If depolarisation is initiated from somewhere other than the sinoatrial node it may have a significant effect on cardiac contraction, or indeed its ability to contract at all. The mechanical contraction of the left ventricle ejects blood into the arteries and this results in a palpable pulse each time. Thus what can be detected by feeling a patients pulse is a direct measure of what is happening to the left ventricle.

Pulses

In a dental surgery setting there are two pulses that can be detected easily. The radial pulse is located at the wrist and should be taken as shown in *Figure 2.2*. It is not advisable to take this pulse using your thumb as this has a pulse of its own and it may then be your own pulse you are feeling.

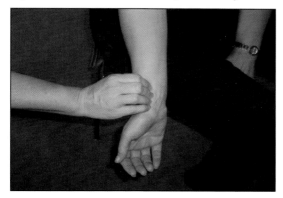

Figure 2.2 Taking the radial pulse.

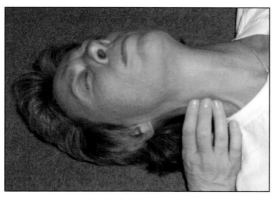

Figure 2.3 Taking the carotid pulse.

The radial pulse is a peripheral pulse, and in a medical emergency the patient may have gone into peripheral shutdown as previously described, therefore it is more reliable to take a central pulse using the common carotid artery as shown in *Figure 2.3*.

In infants the neck is very short and it is very difficult to detect a carotid pulse accurately and therefore a brachial pulse is taken (*Figure 2.4*).

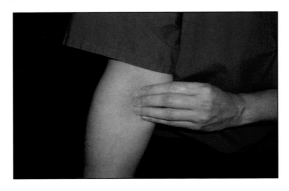

Figure 2.4 Brachial pulse.

By counting the pulse rate over a certain number of seconds it is possible to determine the heart rate, the minimum number of seconds should be 10. For example if the pulse rate over 15 seconds is 20, the heart rate per minute is 20 x 4 = 80 beats per minute (bpm). In a healthy heart the depolarisation occurs regularly, therefore the contraction also occurs regularly, so the pulse should be regular. An irregular pulse is a sign of a significant conduction defect and the patient should be transferred to hospital.

Slow Pulses

This is usually indicative of a slow heart rate and is called a bradycardia. Whilst some athletes can have a slow pulse rate due to their high level of fitness, people with a pulse rate of 50bpm or below may have underlying problems. There are several causes of slow pulse rates and these are shown in *Table 2.1*. The significant one in a dental surgery setting is the one associated with a simple faint.

Fast Pulses

A fast pulse rate reflects a fast heart rate, which is called a tachycardia, and the most common cause of this is anxiety. The ventricles need time to re-fill with blood after each ejection, and if the available filling time is reduced between subsequent contractions because the rate has increased then the volume of blood filling the ventricles will be reduced. It follows, therefore, that the volume of blood at each ejection will be reduced. This will reduce the pulse volume (strength) and make it more difficult to detect. The pulse may be described as a thready or weak pulse. Excluding athletes, a pulse rate of over 150bpm will start to result in a feeling of dizziness, and as the rate increases there will be insufficient blood volume being ejected and the blood pressure will start to fall. There are several causes of fast pulse rates and these are shown in *Table 2.2*.

Table 2.1   Slow pulse rates

Rate and rhythm	Cause	Treatment
50bpm regular	Sinoatrial node transmission blocked and atrio-ventricular node has taken over as pacemaker — 1st degree heartblock	Confirmed by hospital — no treatment usually needed
45-55bpm irregular	Block somewhere in conducting pathway — 2nd degree heartblock	Confirmed by hospital — may require treatment
30-35bpm regular	Transmission between atria and ventricles completely blocked — 3rd degree heartblock. Ventricles have taken over pacemaker	Admission to hospital and cardiac pacemaker fitted
35-45bpm regular	Vaso-vagal syncope (faint)	Increase venous return by lying flat and elevating legs, rate will increase

Table 2.2   Fast pulse rates

Rate and rhythm	Cause	Treatment
100-170bpm regular	Sinus tachycardia — normal heart function but stimulus from central nervous system increasing rate as a result of fear, excitement, etc	Reduce/withdraw stimulus
120-150bpm irregular	Abnormal conduction originating from the atria — usually atrial fibrillation	Confirmed by hospital — may require treatment
150-170bpm regular	Abnormal firing focus above the ventricles (SVTs)	Patient will know if they have SVTs and how to stop them
150-190bpm regular	Ventricular tachycardia, abnormal focus firing in the ventricles, may lead to cardiac arrest	Urgent hospital admission

Cardiac Arrest

Cardiac arrest is a situation in which there is no discernible cardiac output and thus there is no detectable pulse. An immediate priority is to try to compensate for this by instigating manual external compression of the heart. Cardiac compressions (or massage) will force the blood out of the left ventricle and into the circulation (this procedure is covered in Chapter 4). If a cardiac arrest is to be reversed accurate diagnosis and treatment of the cause is essential and therefore it is important to understand the potential causes and what management options there are. There are two broad categories of causation for cardiac arrest. One could be loosely termed electrical misfires, and occurs when the heart muscle is capable of co-ordinated contraction but is getting the wrong electrical stimuli; there is a problem with the conduction system. The other cause is mechanical problems in which there is a problem with the ability of the cardiac muscles to contract, irrespective of what the conduction system is telling it to do.

Electrical misfires

There are two of these — pulseless ventricular tachycardia and ventricular fibrillation. These conditions need to be treated with defibrillation (described later)

Pulseless Ventricular Tachycardia (VT)
A single abnormal focus in the ventricles begins depolarising at an extremely rapid rate. As the conduction pathway cannot stop firing when it is initiated, the 'domino effect' described earlier produces rapid and poorly effective ventricular contraction. There may be sufficient time between contractions for partial ventricular filling so initially there may be a pulse associated with VT, but as the rate increases there will be no filling and therefore no blood ejected into the circulation. The electrical trace will show a fast regular broad complex pattern (*Figure 2.5*).

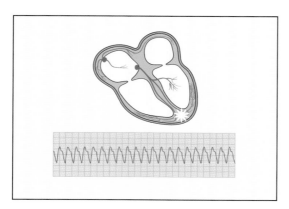

Figure 2.5 Ventricular tachycardia.

Ventricular Fibrillation (VF)

Fibrillation of the ventricles occurs when multiple different electrical foci arise within the heart muscle and begin firing in an indiscriminate pattern. Each foci will produce an initiation of contraction which is then interfered with by the next one. The result is an uncoordinated and ineffective muscle contractions; this is colloquially described as a *bag of worms*. As the muscle is wriggling instead of contracting there will be no cardiac output. The electrical trace will show irregular disordered activity (*Figure 2.6*).

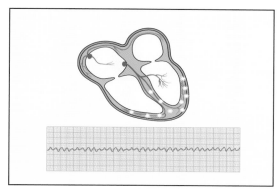

Figure 2.6 Ventricular fibrillation.

Mechanical problems

There are two categories of mechanical causes of cardiac arrest, and they are asytole and pulseless electrical activity (PEA). These are descriptive terms based on what can be seen as an electrical trace.

In asystole there is no evidence of any electrical activity at all, and in PEA the trace can mimic anything including a normal rhythm but there is no cardiac output. If the conducting system is functioning correctly then the heart muscle should contract but there are certain situations that prevent this happening.

The events that might give rise to asystole or PEA may be reversible, and so basic life support is instituted and continued until a potential cause is identified and, if possible, addressed. There are eight broad categories that these causes are grouped into and they are described as the four Hs and four Ts.

The Four Hs:

- **Hypothermia**. Mammalian muscles are designed to function at normal body temperature, as the temperature falls the enzyme systems within the muscle cease to function effectively and the muscle becomes incapable of further contraction unless the temperature is raised. Thus if a person has fallen into freezing water the heart muscle will become incapable of further contraction and they will effectively have a cardiac arrest. If they are re-warmed the muscle will become capable of contracting again.

- **Hypovolaemia**. As stated previously the amount of blood ejected from the heart depends on the amount going into it, if there is a sudden loss of blood volume then the volume in the circulation drops dramatically. Loss of volume may be genuine due to a bleed from major trauma, or effective due to the water component being lost from the circulation because of leaky capillaries as in anaphylaxis. If the circulating blood volume is restored, for example by fluid or blood replacement, then the cardiac output will be re-established.

- **Hypoxia**. No muscle tissue can function without an adequate supply of oxygen, if the heart muscle does not have this it will not work, and hence there will be no cardiac output. If the oxygenation is restored it may recover and begin to function again.

- **Hypo/hyper electrolytes**. There are several chemical compounds that are essential for muscle function, e.g. potassium. These need to be present within fairly fine tolerance limits; too little is as detrimental as too much. If the ideal concentration of potassium is not achieved then the myocardium will not function. If the cause can be identified and rectified then the muscle will resume normal functioning.

The Four Ts:

- **Tamponade**. The heart is enclosed in a strong fibrous pericardial sack, if the patient suffers penetrating chest trauma, such as a stabbing and this results in a bleed within the pericardial sack, then the heart will become compressed due to external pressure. Despite having the ability to contract it is unable to do so. If the pressure is released by removing the blood, then normal function will resume.

- **Tension pneumothorax**. When one of the lungs leaks air into the chest then the lung will collapse under the pressure and that side of the chest will fill with air that has no route of escape. This will cause the pressure within the chest to rise and will push the heart over to the opposite side. This will directly apply pressure onto the muscle, effectively 'squeezing' it so it can no longer contract. If the air is released then the pressure is removed normal myocardial contraction can be resumed.

- **Toxins**. When drugs are taken that affect muscular contraction, then a cardiac arrest can occur. An example of this would be curare, which paralyzes muscle tissue. The only treatment is to identify the drug and supply an antidote.

- **Thromboembolic**. When a clot forms in one or more of the coronary arteries that supply the heart muscle the supply of oxygenated blood to that part of the myocardium will cease and the heart muscle will die. If the clot can be eradicated then the blood supply will be re-established and the muscle may recover and begin to function again.

Paediatric Cardiac Arrest

This is incredibly rare and is most likely to be due to hypoxia. An infant is defined as being in cardiac arrest when the pulse rate is 60bpm or below, and cardiac compressions should be commenced.

CHAPTER 3

Fundamentals of the Nervous System

The body's nervous system can be considered as the instruction and communication network; it is also a control centre for most of the body's organ systems and process. The nervous system is a complex and interlinked system and a detailed discussion of its structure and functions is out with the scope of this book. A basic understanding of the main components of the nervous system, however, is helpful in the management of medical emergencies. This chapter gives a brief resume of the nervous system to facilitate the acquisition of this knowledge.

The nervous system can be divided into two main components, based on the individual functions that these areas are responsible for:

The Central Nervous System (CNS)
This is comprised of the brain and spinal cord. The brain is the most complicated part of the nervous system. The CNS generates messages and instructions and these are ultimately transmitted to the relevant organ systems, via the spinal cord, and these are known as efferent impulses. The CNS also receives and processes information received from the various organs of the body through the spinal cord and these are known as afferent, or sensory, impulses. The CNS is responsible for the integration of all nervous activity.

The Peripheral Nervous System (PNS)
This is comprised of the nerve fibres that leave the CNS and travel out to all the peripheral areas of the body. They are composed of both efferent and afferent nerves thus providing a two way communication system. Part of the PNS is under voluntary control and part is automatically controlled by the brain. The PNS is therefore divided into two discrete systems, dependent upon voluntary and involuntary control.

• The cranial nerves and the spinal nerves which are under voluntary control. There are 12 pairs of nerves that exit directly from the brain and these are called the cranial nerves and some of these are responsible for the special senses such as sight, hearing and taste. There are also 31 spinal nerves on each side that progressively leave the spinal cord at descending levels to supply the upper and lower limbs and the main trunk of the body.

- The autonomic nervous system (ANS) is an 'involuntary' nervous system and we have no conscious control over it. The ANS controls the heart and other involuntary smooth muscles (for example in the walls of blood vessels, bronchi and in the intestine), secreting glands such as the salivary glands, sweat glands, the endocrine glands, etc. The ANS is subdivided into two parts: the sympathetic and the parasympathetic system. The sympathetic system is responsible for your body's 'fight or flight' reaction. The parasympathetic system looks after the workings of your body during rest and recuperation. It also controls your heart rate and body temperature under normal conditions.

Organs may be supplied predominantly by one division of the ANS or by both the sympathetic and parasympathetic system. When an organ is supplied by both systems they will then have opposing effects and act in a complementary manner. An example of this is the ANS control of the heart, the parasympathetic system will decrease the heart rate but the sympathetic nerve supply will increase the heart rate.

From a resuscitation perspective, the sympathetic system is the more relevant as it becomes active in times of stress and causes an increase in heart rate, dilatation of the bronchi, it diverts the blood away from the digestive system and the skin and diverts it to skeletal muscles, the heart and lungs. When a patient becomes physically 'stressed' during an emergency the typical appearance is to become 'pale and sweaty' due to the effects of the sympathetic nervous system on the skin and sweat glands. The parasympathetic nervous system, however, can be important in a faint as an increase in vagal activity causes the heart rate to slow down considerably and the patient faints (vasovagal attack). *Table 3.1* outlines the supply of the ANS to certain organs and tissues.

What Affects the Nervous System?

Anxiety

The CNS is responsible for processing all the information regarding the persons environment and taking the appropriate action. When an individual becomes stressed and fearful a whole series of responses will be activated over which they have no voluntary control; adrenaline will be produced which is a powerful stimulating hormone and the sympathetic nervous

Table 3.1   The innervation of some tissues with the autonomic nervous system

Organ	Sympathetic activity	Parasympathetic activity
Eye	Dilates pupil	Constricts pupils
Bronchial smooth muscle	Dilates bronchi	Constricts bronchi
Heart	Increases heart rate	Decreases heart rate
Salivary glands and digestive tract	Reduces activity	Increases activity

system will begin to have a direct effect on the heart and lungs. The best way of reducing these effects, which are unhelpful in the dental chair (but are advantageous if you are preparing to run away), is to ensure that the patient's anxiety is reduced as far as possible. If a patient is extremely nervous it may be better to consider treatment with sedation.

Drugs

There are many drugs that can have a direct effect on the nervous system, and some are prescribed specifically for this purpose. Many medicines however, have unwanted side-effects on the CNS so a thorough drugs history is essential. One group of drugs that the patient may not readily admit to taking is recreational drugs, and these can have profound CNS effects. *Table 3.2* gives examples of drugs which may have a direct effect on the nervous system.

Glucose

In common with all the other tissues in the body, nervous tissue requires glucose as a source of energy. As there is no mechanism for glucose to be stored within nerves, correct functioning is entirely dependent on the immediate availability of glucose in the bloodstream, and there can be significant detrimental effects if this level is too high or too low.

Oxygen

The brain is the major user of oxygen and any interruption to an adequate supply will result in confusion, loss of consciousness and ultimately death. Hypoxia of the CNS can either be due to lack of oxygen in the circulating

Table 3.2   Examples of drugs that have an effect on the CNS

Drug	Effect
Alcohol	CNS depressant, impaired concentration and judgement, euphoria, depression
Benzodiazepines (e.g. diazepam, midazolam)	CNS depressant, impaired concentration and judgement
Opioids (e.g morphine, pethidine, heroin)	CNS depressant, lack of concentration, irritability
Amphetamines (e.g. cocaine)	CNS stimulant, mood elevators, can produce paranoia and tactile hallucinations
Hallucinogens (e.g. LSD)	Mimic sympathetic nervous system — pupil dilation, sweating, rapid pulse rate, produces significant hallucinations

blood (this will be because of poor oxygenation in the lungs), or interruption to the CNS blood supply. For example, in the early stages of a respiratory arrest, the CNS has a circulation but the blood is not adequately oxygenated. However, if the blood pressure falls there will be an insufficient blood supply to the CNS and this will result in loss of consciousness; despite the oxygen saturation levels of the blood being satisfactory. Similarly in a stroke (CVA) the blood vessels supplying part of the brain are blocked — occluded — and the deprivation of oxygenated blood results in tissue death.

Trauma

This can either be direct trauma to a part of the CNS or peripheral nerves, e.g. spinal cord injury, which will permanently affect the transmission of the nervous impulses, or indirect trauma from pressure. A tumour or a bleed within the brain can press against the nerves and prevent them working effectively — this effect can sometimes be reversed when the cause of the pressure is removed.

Disease

There are many disease processes that can affect nervous system, but the ones most relevant to dentistry are epilepsy, Parkinson's disease, multiple sclerosis and motor neurone disease. It is important to realise that these patients already have a compromised nervous system. Epilepsy is also important because it can present as a medical emergency. This is usually caused by an abnormal focus in the brain that starts to send out impulses in an uncontrolled and disordered manner. These impulses are not related to physiological needs. The efferent nerves then conduct these impulses to the muscles in the limbs, producing the classic jerking movements of a seizure. The symptoms will depend, however, upon the part of the brain that is affected. Epilepsy is discussed in more detail as a medical emergency in chapter 12.

Assessment of the Central Nervous System

There would never be an indication for a full assessment of the CNS in a dental surgery setting, but there are some simple tests that can be carried out that will provide valuable information about the patient.

Level of consciousness

This has traditionally been assessed in a hospital setting using the 'Glasgow coma scale', where three separate responses are given a numerical score, and then the score is added up. The maximum available score is 15 (*Table 3.3*)

The difficulty with this assessment is that it is difficult to use and overly complicated for a dental surgery setting. The more commonly used assessment of consciousness is called Alert/Verbal/Painful/Unresponsive (AVPU). This is used to describe the patients overall state of consciousness; alert; vocal response; pain/pressure response and unresponsive. The AVPU classification is explained more fully in *Table 3.4*.

Pupil responses

The pupil of the eye is a circular opening, or aperture, at the centre of the iris and allows light through to the lens of the eye. The iris is a muscle formed by a series of ringed fibres that allow it to dilate or constrict depending on the amount of light that is entering it. This is a reflex reaction with no voluntary control, and if a light is shone into one eye the pupils of both eyes will immediately constrict. If a persons pupils do not constrict in this synchronous manner it is a sign of CNS depression or pathology of some kind.

In a dental surgery it is a simple task to shine the dental light into a patient's eyes and measure the response, the possible outcomes are given in *Table 3.5*. It is also of relevance to remember that a patient who has opioids in their bloodstream will have constricted pupils.

Table 3.3   The Glasgow Coma Scale

Eyes open	Score	Verbal response	Score	Motor response	Score
				Obeys commands	6
		Orientated	5	Localises pain	5
Spontaneously	4	Confused	4	Withdrawal from pain	4
To speech	3	Innapropriate words	3	Flexion to pain	3
To pain	2	Incomprensible sounds	2	Extension to pain	2
Never	I	Silent	I	No motor response	I

Table 3.4   Alert/verbal/painful/unresponsive

Level chosen	Patient response
A	Patient is awake and alert, responds directly and logically to question, talking to you
V	Patient only responds when spoken to, response may be slightly incoherent, no spontaneous conversation
P	Patient unresponsive unless touched with pressure or pain, e.g. will pull hand away when squeezed. No conversation response
U	Patient is completely unresponsive whatever the stimulus

Table 3.5 **Pupil response to light**

Response	Cause
Unilateral constriction only	Possible cerebrovascular accident (CVA)
Slow bilateral response	CNS depression
Pupils very constricted initially (i.e. not light dependant)	Under influence of drugs
Fixed and dilated — non responsive	Patient has had cardiac arrest

Section 2

Emergency Procedures

CHAPTER 4

Basic Life Support

All healthcare professionals must be capable of providing basic life support (BLS) to an adequate standard. The only way to achieve this is to attend a formal BLS course with practical hands-on skill stations using simulators to ensure that the necessary techniques have been mastered, and these courses should be attended on an annual basis to ensure skill maintenance. There are guidelines published by the Resuscitation Council (UK) which are updated approximately every 2 years and all practitioners should consult the website (www.resus.org.uk) on a regular basis to ensure they are thoroughly familiar with the current guidance. It is also good practice to hold regular scenario training within the dental surgery so that practice teams get a chance to refine and hone their skills on a more frequent basis.

The principle of BLS is to provide:

- Artificial respiration to a patient who is not breathing spontaneously
- To maintain a circulation by chest compressions in patients who haveno spontaneous circulation.

The principle of cardiac compressions is that the heart is squeezed by the downward pressure, forcing blood out of the ventricles and into the circulation. When this pressure is released the ventricles refill by suction and this blood is expelled by the next compression. It is therefore important to remember that the downward pressure exerted must be sufficient to force the blood out, and that the pressure must be released completely after each compression to allow the heart to refill.

When a person has a cardiorespiratory arrest the provision of BLS is not a cure, it is a method of continuing to supply oxygenated blood to the brain whilst any contributing factors and cause for the arrest can be identified and reversed if possible. It is best described as being part of the 'chain of survival' which is a term used to describe a sequence of events that provide the best opportunity for a patient to survive following a catastrophic event (*Figure 4.1*).

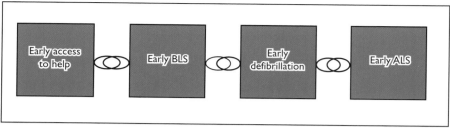

Figure 4.1 The chain of survival. Adapted from Laerdal Medical Ltd.

The BLS Sequence

In a dental surgery a patient already has the first part of the chain in place, as they have early access to help. A collapsed patient should always be approached in the same way:

- Ensure that it is safe to approach the patient. Whilst the dental surgery is usually a safe environment it is still good practice to check for electrical cables and potential 'trip' hazards
- Assess the patient's response by calling them by name (if known) and asking loudly if they are all right, also shake them gently and firmly to see if there is any response. At this stage it is useful to call for help from your work colleagues.

If there is evidence of a response at this point, then an ABCDE assessment must be instigated and the patient needs to be placed in the recovery position to enable airway protection (*Figure 4.2a-d)*).

The recommended procedure to place a patient into the recovery position is as follows (assuming the patient is lying on their back):

1. Remove any items of personal equipment which have the potential to cause harm, such as glasses, and remember to check the patient's pockets for keys, pens. etc.
2. Kneel at the patient's side and position the arm nearest to you into the position shown (*Figure 4.2a*)
3. Reach across the patient and bring their other arm across their chest, placing their hand against their cheek (*Figure 4.2b*)
4. Bend the opposite leg so that the foot is flat on the floor and the knee is raised (*Figure 4.2c*)
5. Ensuring that the patients neck is supported roll the patient towards you (*Figure 4.2d*).

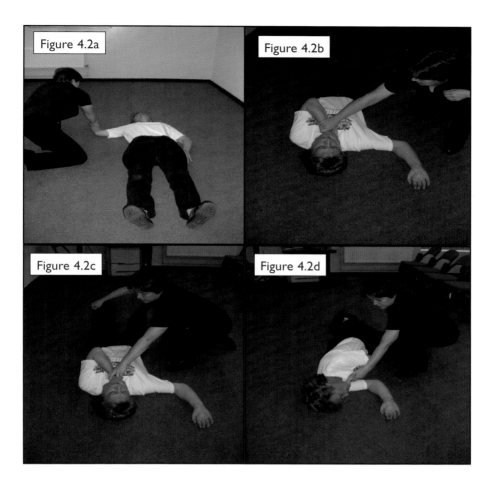

Figure 4.2a
Figure 4.2b
Figure 4.2c
Figure 4.2d

Important points to remember are to continue to monitor ABCDE the whole time, and if the patient has been in this position for 30 minutes it is necessary to turn them onto the opposite side to prevent compression bruising.

- If there is no response from the patient then this will be a commencement of a formal ABCDE assessment so the first thing to check is the airway, as described in chapter two
- If the airway is clear then breathing is assessed — if breathing is present then the patient should be placed in the recovery position, if not then check for a pulse or any signs of life. This is usually done together as a synchronous breathing and pulse check
- If there is no breathing and no pulse then telephone for an ambulance

to ensure help is on its way and cardiopulmonary resuscitation must be commenced immediately. Within a dental surgery setting other team members can be summoned and duties delegated to each member
- Chest compressions and ventilations should be started. The ratio of compressions to ventilations will vary depending upon age. In adults the ratio is 30 compressions followed by 2 ventilations — 30:2
- BLS should continue until help arrives or until the rescuer is too tired to continue. Providing chest compressions is extremely tiring and it is recommended that team members take turns every two to three minutes to prevent exhaustion.

Chest Compressions

Adults

The rate of compressions should be 100 per minute and the chest should be compressed to a depth of 4-5cm. Thirty compressions are followed by two ventilations.

For chest compressions to be effective the patient must be positioned flat on their back against a hard surface. The floor is ideal, but a dental chair can be positioned flat enough and is rigid enough to withstand the force of the compressions. It is not necessary to move the patient out of the dental chair. If any movement of the patient is necessary to change their position care must be taken to protect the cervical spine so the neck must be supported at all times during the movement. Chest compressions are best undertaken whilst you are standing at the side of the patient, adjacent to their chest, or kneeling if the patient is on the floor. The following is a guide on how to undertake chest compressions:

- Place the heel of one hand in the centre of the patient's chest, and position the heel of the other hand directly over it
- Either extend or interlock your fingers to ensure they are not touching the ribs
- Lean forwards so that your arms are straight and your shoulders are directly over your arms (*Figure 4.3*)
- Using a rocking motion from your hips apply sufficient downward force onto the sternum to depress it 4-5 cm
- Allow the chest to recoil completely without moving your hands and then apply the next compression.

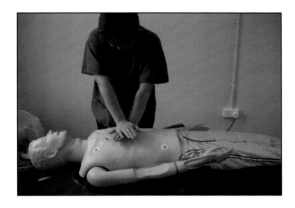

Figure 4.3 Correct position for chest compressions

After each set of 30 chest compressions supply two effective ventilations. It is acknowledged that some rescuers may be unwilling to undertake mouth to mouth ventilations and in this case the head should be positioned so the airway is open, e.g. by a 'head tilt/chin lift' and the compressions are supplied continually. There will be a small amount of room air drawn into the lungs by the compressions alone.

Children

The ratio of chest compressions to breathes in children is:

- Aged 0-8 years 15:2
- Aged over 8 years 30:2

Children over the age of 8 years are treated in the same way as adults, and the rate of compressions is always 100 per minute irrespective of the age of the child. There main difference with providing cardiac compressions in children is the hand position and depth of compressions, and how many compressions that are given before ventilation.

Infants (under 1 year old)
Encircle the chest with your hands and apply the compressions using both thumbs and depress the chest by 1-2 cm, as shown in *Figure 4.4*.

Alternatively, use two fingers of one hand placed just below the inter nipple line, as shown in *Figure 4.5*.

Children aged 1-8 years
The compressions should be administered with one hand only with a compression depth of 2-3 cm. The hand position is shown in *Figure 4.6*, and in older children the heel of the hand would be used.

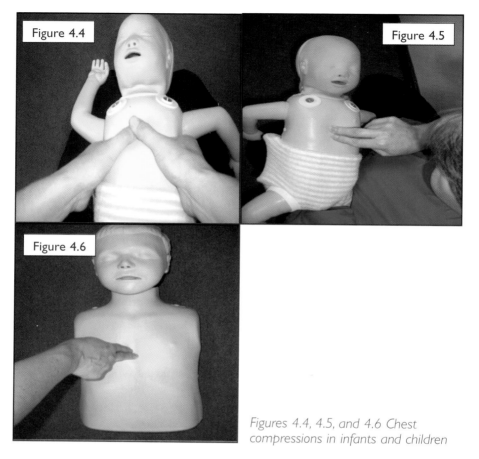

Figures 4.4, 4.5, and 4.6 Chest compressions in infants and children

Ventilations and Rescue Breaths

This was covered in detail in Chapter 1. In adults it is felt to be more important to commence the cardiac compressions before the rescue breaths.

In children, however, it is essential that breaths are administered before cardiac compressions are initiated. If a child is unresponsive and there is no breathing then five rescue breathes are given before checking for a pulse. If no pulse is detectable then CPR is instigated at 15:2 for one minute before leaving the patient to call the paramedics.

The sequence of events is therefore slightly different in children and adults and both are summarised in *Figure 4.7* and *Figure 4.8*.

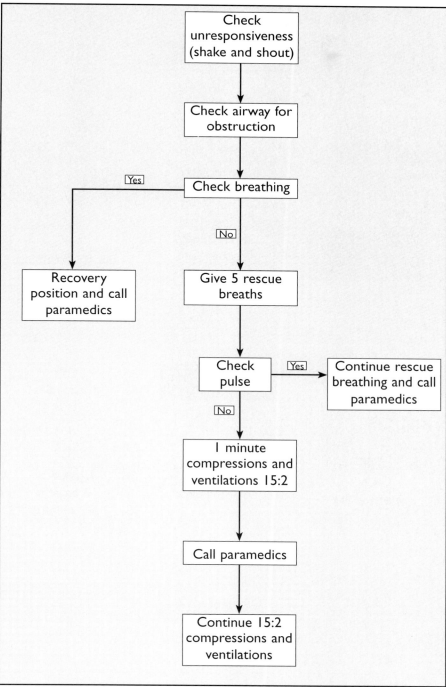

Figure 4.7 Sequence summary – paediatric basic life support. Adapted from the Resuscitation Council UK.

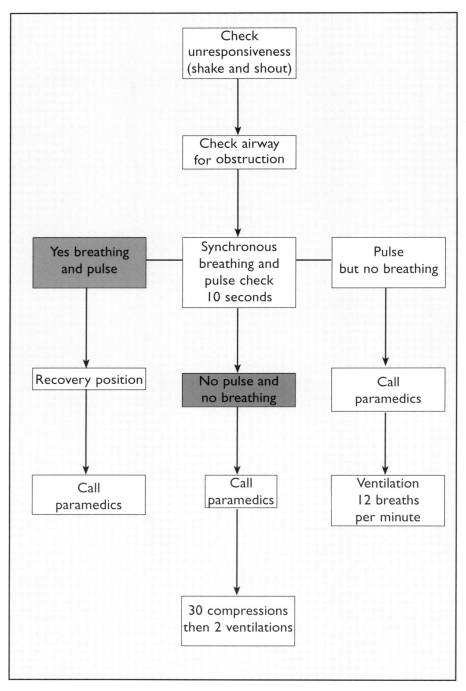

Figure 4.8 Sequence summary – adult basic life support. Adapted from the Resuscitation Council UK

CHAPTER 5

Defibrillation

When a patient has a cardiac arrest the outcome is usually poor and therefore any action that can be taken to improve the chances of survival is worthwhile. As stated previously, good quality basic life support (BLS) will help to maintain some oxygenated circulation to the brain, but it is only a temporary measure until the cause of the arrest can be established and reversed if possible — BLS is a holding operation. The causes of a cardiac arrest were discussed in chapter 2, and these were divided into two generic categories: 'electrical' misfires and 'mechanical' causes. Defibrillation is an effective method of treating and reversing the electrical problem but has no relevance in the treatment of the mechanical causes.

Cardiac arrest can be caused by rapid but ineffective electrical activity. This is called pulseless ventricular tachycardia (VT) or ventricular fibrillation (VF), and in both of these conditions the nervous impulses travelling through the conduction system are originating too quickly and in the wrong places — the myocardium is misfiring and the contractions are uncontrolled. The cardiac muscle is capable of conducting electricity and should be able to function normally again if these aberrant impulses can be stopped. During pulseless VT or VF the heart muscle is contracting rapidly and erratically and will quickly become exhausted and eventually will stop contracting, therefore, time is a vital factor if the outcome is to be improved. The chances of successful treatment of a pulseless VT/VF arrest decrease by 7-10% per minute as shown *Figure 5.1*.

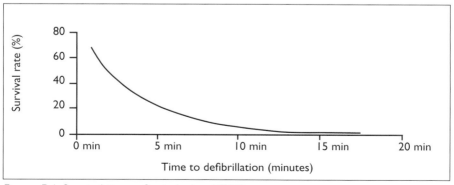

Figure 5.1 Survival time of a pulseless VT/VF arrest.
Information source: Resuscitation Council UK

How does Defibrillation Work?

One way to understand the basic principles of how and why a defibrillator works is to use an analogy of a hysterical person in a room. If you entered a room and a person was running about in hysterics then you know that the person is functioning but in an uncontrolled and disorganised way. If you go to them and hit them across the face you will be effectively delivering a *short sharp shock* that will momentarily stun them, hopefully they will then recover control and function properly. This is the type of response you want when you defibrillate cardiac muscle. A normal cardiac impulse originates from the sino-atrial node, the body's natural pacemaker, and this electrical activity spreads down the conducting system to the cardiac muscle, causing the myocardium to depolarise and thus contract. In a VF arrest the muscle fibres are all contracting in a random and disorganised way. If a large direct electrical current is applied to the whole area of cardiac muscle at the same time it will all contract simultaneously and then enter the 'refractory' phase (i.e. no activity is possible for a short period of time). The first area to recover from this refractory phase is the sino-atrial node, which will then discharge through the conducting pathways as normal and the cardiac muscle will contract in an organised and functional way.

What is a defibrillator?

A defibrillator is the machine that produces a large electrical shock that can be applied to a the myocardium. Early defibrillators were heavy cumbersome machines that had to be set manually by the operator to deliver a specified charge or amount of electricity. The charge was delivered through paddles that were held manually against a patient's chest whilst delivering the shock. These defibrillators could only be used by highly trained personnel. The introduction of automated external defibrillators (AEDs) has simplified this process and improved safety so that they can be used in settings outside of the hospital.

An AED has two adhesive pads that are attached to the patient's chest, the machine monitors the arrest rhythm and if it recognises an electrical misfire (VF or pulseless VT) it will charge up ready to deliver a shock at the correct energy level. When the operator is satisfied that it is safe for a shock to be delivered, they press a button on the machine and the shock is delivered through adhesive pads placed onto the chest. The machine has voice prompts which inform the operator what is happening and will advise whether a shock is indicated or not.

There are two types of AED; monophasic ones are the older type and they deliver a shock in one direction only, while bi-phasic machines have now been developed which actually deliver a shock in each direction between the pads (two small smacks as opposed to one big smack!). The bi-phasic machines are lighter and smaller and are found on aircraft and in railway stations and shopping centres. They are simple and easy to use and the operator cannot override the machine. It is impossible to deliver a shock when it is not appropriate.

How do you use an AED?

There is considerable discussion at the moment as to whether defibrillation should be taught as part of BSL as it is a crucial step in the chain of survival, and there is no doubt that the survival rates from out of hospital arrests have increased since the widespread availability of AEDs. The Resuscitation Council UK has recommended that all dental practices have an AED on the premises. However all healthcare professionals who wish to use a defibrillator must be trained in their safe use. One way to do this is to attend a Resuscitation Council Immediate Life Support (ILS) course.

Step 1

When a cardiac arrest has been diagnosed commence BLS and send for the AED (*Figure 5.2a-d*). It needs to be removed from its case and switched on — they are usually battery powered although some may need to be connected to the mains supply. There will be a set of adhesive pads with a connector at one end which needs to be plugged into the machine — a voice prompt will remind you of this and it is impossible to connect them the wrong way round.

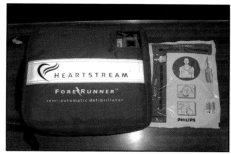

Figure 5.2a The defibrillator package.

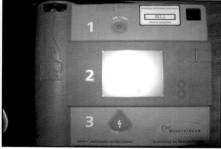

Figure 5.2b The machine.

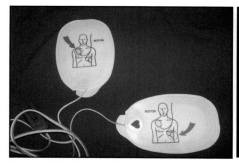

Figure 5.2c The pads.

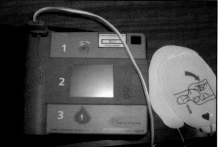

Figure 5.2d Pads connected.

Step 2

The pads need to be applied to the patient's bare chest as shown in *Figure 5.3*. There are diagrams on each pad to demonstrate the correct positioning, however if the pads are placed the wrong way round it does not matter as long as they are in the correct position on the chest. It is not worth wasting valuable time repositioning them. There are several crucial points to be considered during this step:

- The pads must be pressed firmly onto the skin with no creases or air trapped underneath
- The chest skin must be clean and dry
- The presence of chest hair will reduce the pad contact so it should be cut with scissors prior to pad placement. Cutting with scissors is preferable to shaving as any nicks or cuts will produce bleeding and fluid of any sort will reduce the effective charge delivery. Also time is vital so it is not worth waiting to locate a razor
- It is inadvisable to place a pad over breast tissue so it may be necessary to place a pad more laterally in female patients
- There must be no metal in contact with, or near to the pads, e.g underwired bras, etc.
- CPR needs to be ongoing whilst this is taking place.

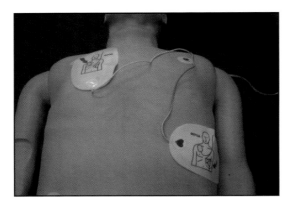

Figure 5.3 The pads in place.

Step 3

The machine will begin analysing the heart rhythm and will remind you of this with a voice prompt; whilst this is taking place CPR is temporarily halted as the machine will not be able to assess the rhythm accurately whilst the patient is moving. The defibrillator will then advise whether a shock is necessary, it will voice prompt either '*shock advised*' or '*no shock advised*', if the latter is stated then the arrest is not one of the shockable rhythms and basic CPR must be continued.

Step 4

If a shock is advised then the machine will begin to emit a noise as it charges up ready to deliver the shock. When it is fully charged a light will flash on a button which will need to be depressed to actually deliver the shock. The operator is responsible for pressing this button and there is a vital safety protocol which must be carried out first:

- No one must be in direct contact with the patient otherwise they will receive a shock also
- No one should be in indirect contact (e.g. touching the dental chair) or in contact with any fluid that may be around the patient
- The oxygen must be at least 1 meter away because it is highly flammable and could explode
- The operator should check all of the above and say in a loud voice '*Oxygen away and stand clear*'
- The shock is then delivered.

Step 5

Once the shock has been delivered CPR is resumed immediately and continued for 2 minutes until the machine voice prompts for the next rhythm analysis. The machines are designed to time these intervals and there will be another voice prompt when it is time to re-analyse the heart rhythm.

These steps are repeated in sequence for as long as the machine advises a shock is necessary. There is no necessity to carry out a pulse check unless prompted by the AED, and CPR is continued throughout except when the machine is analysing the rhythm and when the shock is actually being delivered. The shock level is expressed in joules and is preset on the machine.

Children

It is extremely rare for a child to have an arrest with a shockable rhythm. Should defibrillation be necessary for a paediatric arrest and the child is aged 8 or over, then adult defibrillation pads and machines can be used. There are specialised paediatric AEDs and pads available but they would be unlikely to be present in a dental surgery.

Figure 5.4 overleaf shows an algorithm for AED defibrillation.

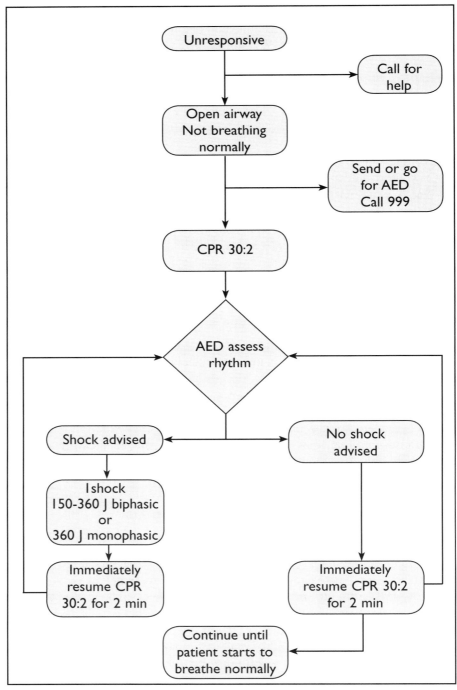

Figure 5.4 Algorithm for AED defibrillation. Reproduced with permission of the Resuscitation Council UK

CHAPTER 6

Emergency Drugs and Routes of Administration

All dental surgeries must have an emergency drug box on the premises to be available for use in the event of a medical emergency. The range and type of drugs that are recommended for use can vary depending on the authority consulted. However, a more uniform approach is now developing between the various bodies that issue guidance — this will reduce the inconsistencies and conflict that has existed in past recommendations.

The current recommendations from the British National Formulary, the Resuscitation Council (UK) and the Scottish Dental Clinical Effectiveness Programme are shown in *Table 6.1* overleaf. It should be remembered that with the introduction of new evidence this list is likely to be updated over time.

It is of paramount importance that all staff should be familiar with the emergency drugs that the practice carries and understand the indications for their use. There can be considerable variations in the way a drug may be packaged for use — this is called the presentation. It is essential that all staff examine the presentation of the drugs in their emergency drug kit to ensure they are familiar with preparing each drug for delivery in an emergency situation. A clinical emergency should not be the first time you have prepared the drug. The best way to develop and maintain competency in preparing emergency drug preparations is to actually practice using out-of-date products. This will allow all members of the dental team have the opportunity to become familiar with the required tasks and in the event of an emergency can help to reduce panic, save time and increase confidence. Although some staff members may be reticent about actually administering some of the drugs it is still worthwhile practising drug preparation because any member of the dental team may be called upon to help. Teamwork is vital in the successful management of an emergency.

There are also several different methods by which drugs can be administered, and sometimes the same drug can be given in different ways, so again it is worth training as a team to gain an understanding of the different routes of administration for the drugs carried in the surgery.

The following sections describe the possible routes of administration and discuss the different forms of preparation currently available, followed by a description of each individual drug with the indications for its use, its mode of action, the time it takes to be effective and the routes of administration.

Table 6.1 **Current recommendations for emergency drugs required for a dental surgery from three different authoritative bodies**

British National Formulary No55 March 2008	Resuscitation Council www.resus.org.uk (2006)	Scottish Dental Clinical Effectiveness Programme www.scottishdental.org/cep
Oxygen	Oxygen (size D) cylinder	Two size D or one size E
Salbutamol inhaler	Salbutamol inhaler	Salbutamol inhaler
Adrenaline (epinephrine) (1:1000)	Adrenaline (epinephrine) (1:1000)	Adrenaline (epinephrine) (1:1000)
Glucagon	Glucagon	Glucagon
Aspirin dispersible tablets	Aspirin dispersible tablets	Aspirin dispersible tablets
GTN spray or tablets	GTN spray	GTN spray
Glucose, oral or buccal	Glucose, oral or buccal	Glucose, oral or buccal
Mizadolam, buccal liquid 10mg/ml or injection (2mg/ml or 5mg/ml) for buccal route	Midazolam, buccal liquid 10mg/ml or 5mg/ml for buccal or intranasal route	Midazolam 10mg/ml buccal route

Possible Routes of Administration

The more quickly the drug reaches the correct concentration in the blood the more quickly it will become effective. The time taken for a drug to be successful will depend, in part, on how it is administered. This will influence its rate of absorption and the time taken to get to the main site of action. The various methods of drug administration that are used in the management of medical emergencies in the dental surgery are summarised in *Table 6.2*. Drugs may be absorbed through the skin, the alveoli of the lungs, and the gastro-intestinal tract. They can be injected directly into the blood, or can be deposited in areas of high blood flow so that they can be absorbed quickly and effectively via the capillary network. Some drugs can be administered by several different methods, others may be ineffective if given by an

Table 6.2   The different methods of drug administration

Route of administration	Absorption time
Intravenous	20–60 seconds
Inhalation	1–5 minutes

Transmucosal
    Sublingual
    Buccal
    Intranasal
	
	1–2 minutes
	1–5 minutes
	5–15 minutes

Intramuscular	5–15 minutes
Subcutaneous	15–20 minutes
Oral	0.5–2 hours

inappropriate route — many medicines cannot be taken orally as stomach acids inactivate them.

Oral

This is a familiar route that is used for many medicines, for example taking a paracetamol for a headache. Drugs administered by this route will either be in the form of a solid preparation (a tablet or capsule), a liquid, or a dispersible preparation that is dissolved in water. The problem with using an oral route of administration in an emergency situation is the time it takes for the drug to be absorbed into the circulation and become effective. The preparation has to be absorbed across the stomach or intestinal to enter the blood stream. When the stomach is full this can take hours, but if it is empty absorption can occur in as little as 30 minutes. It is no surprise therefore that there is an element of unpredictability in estimating the onset of action of a drug given orally. Drugs used in resuscitation are only administered orally when immediate action is not required.

Transmucosal

Some drug preparations have been designed to cross the thin lining of mucosa in various areas of the body, typically the sublingual and buccal mucosa of the mouth, the nasal mucosa and the rectal mucosa. Once the drug has penetrated the mucosal surface it is rapidly absorbed and distributed by the large network of capillaries present in these areas. Absorbtion across the oral mucosa can produce adequate blood levels after just a few minutes. Absorption across the rectal mucosa can take up to 15 minutes.

Buccal and sublingual preparations are available as either sprays (giving a metered dose per spray), a dissolvable tablet or 'wafer' or lozenge (which is placed under the tongue or against the cheek and allowed to dissolve), a tube of gel or liquid which should be deposited into the buccal sulcus, or around the oral mucosa.

Rectal preparations can be in the form of a suppository or pre-prepared tube with an applicator which allows a liquid form of the drug to be administered by the rectal route. There is no need for dentists to administer emergency drugs by the rectal route.

Nasal preparations can be administered by an atomisation device (*Figure 6.1*) that is attached to the end of a syringe and squirted into the nose.

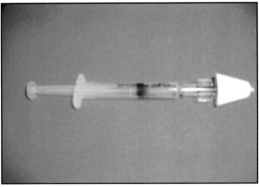

Figure 6.1 Nasal atomisation device attached to a 1ml syringe

Inhalation

The absorption and effect of drugs administered by this route is rapid, around 1 to 5 minutes, as the thinness of the alveoli and capillary endothelium allows rapid transfer into the blood. Medicines administered by this route can be given:

* As a gas
* Inhaler where the patient actuates the device which administers a 'puff' of the drug (usually in the form of a fine powder) which is inhaled directly
* Nebulised (a vapourised mist of fine droplets of liquid drug in a stream of oxygen or air).

A vapouriser or nebuliser is a small device that is attached in-between an air or oxygen tube and a mask (*Figures 6.2a* and *6.2b*). The top of the nebuliser is removed and the contents of the nebule poured into the base of the nebuliser, and this is connected directly to the oxygen air supply and the mask. A measured quantity of the drug is mixed with the air or oxygen on each inhalation.

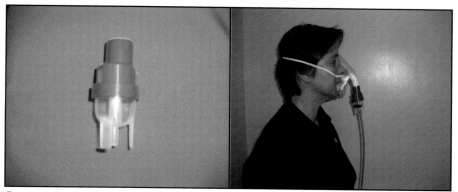

Figure 6.2a A nebuliser   *Figure 6.2b A nebuliser in position*

Injectable Routes

Certain emergency drugs have to be administered by injection, and three commonly used routes include:

- Intravenous (IV)
- Intramuscular (IM)
- Subcutaneous (SC).

In dental practice it is only likely that the IM route would be used in the management of medical emergencies. One exception would be the use of IV flumazenil (the benzodiazepine antagonist) that may be used to reverse oversedation; in this situation the patient will have an IV cannula already in place. The presentations of all drugs for injection vary considerably and therefore the preparation of these for injection requires practice.

Intravenous

This method relies on getting access to a vein and injecting the drug directly into the bloodstream, the onset of action of the drug is very rapid — 20 to 30 seconds. It requires considerable skill to use this technique and there are several potential complications. It is necessary to attend a specific course in order to learn how to gain intravenous access and it is not intended to cover this route in detail here. The only emergency drug that must be given by this route is epinephrine (adrenaline) used in cardiac arrest which most dental surgeries do not have in their emergency drug boxes, if it is available it will again require considerable skill to administer and this should be left to the paramedics.

Intramuscular

This method relies on depositing a specified amount of a drug in a liquid formulation (no more than 5 ml) directly into a large muscle (*Figure 6.7*). The drugs will be absorbed rapidly, over 5 to 15 minutes, into the blood stream. Skeletal muscle has a rich blood supply. The usual sites chosen are either the deltoid muscle in the upper arm, or the outer thigh. It has been suggested that the tongue is a suitable muscle to use but the authors do not recommend this due to the possible complications of bleeding and swelling. In an emergency situation there is rarely a need to remove clothing because the needle tip is quite fine (therefore unlikely to carry cloth fibres into the injection site) and the clothing layers are usually quite thin. The administration of an IM injection is very simple:

- Use the non-injecting hand to 'pinch' the muscle and lift it slightly
- Insert the needle quickly to about two thirds of its length into the 'pinched' muscle tissue
- Aspirate to ensure the needle tip is not in a blood vessel
- Inject the drug, withdraw the needle and apply a pressure dressing.
- Dispose of the sharp safely.

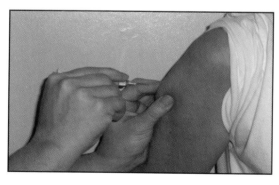

Figure 6.7 An intramuscular injection.

Subcutaneous

This method relies on depositing the drug in the adipose (fatty) tissue just below the skin surface. The rate of absorption is slower that with an IM injection because the blood supply to the adipose layer is not as good as to muscle. The rate of absorption varies from 15 to 20 minutes, and the quantity of solution deposited should be only 1–2 mls. Type I diabetics use this method of administration for their insulin and heparin is also administered by this route. The skin is 'pinched' between the fingers and the needle inserted just below the skin surface, aspirate to ensure a vessel has not been penetrated and then deposit the drug slowly, administration. The skin surface will blanch as the drug is injected. The length of needle required for a SC injection is shorter than that used for an IM injection.

Presentations and preparation

Pre-prepared syringes: These are very simple to use as they are ready for immediate administration, open the container (*Figure 6.3a*), remove the syringe (*Figure 6.3b*), take the cap of the needle (*Figure 6.3c*) and syringe is ready for use (*Figure 6.3d*). The disadvantage of these preparations is that the bung of the syringe may contain latex so the manufacturers details must be carefully checked.

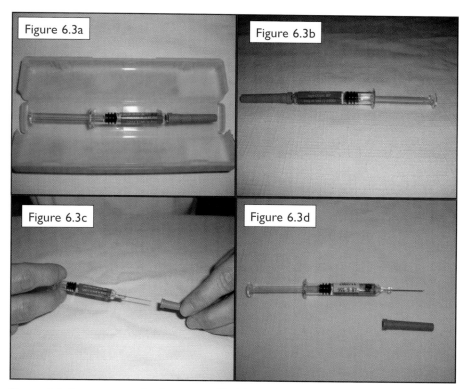

Figure 6.3 Four stages of using a pre-filled hypodermic syringe.

Minijet®️ syringes: This system is used extensively for emergency drugs in hospitals, but in dentistry only adrenaline is presented in this format. Whilst this system is easy to assemble, training is required to assemble the component parts into a fully functioning syringe. The assembly of Minijet® (*Figure 6.4*) is often called the 'flip and tip' system. It consist of two separate components: the delivery system and the pre-prepared drug in a cartridge. This system is latex free. The sequence of actions is as follows:

1. Remove both tubes from the box (*Figure 6.4a*). One tube will be a glass tube, which contains the liquid drug and will have a coloured plastic stopper on the top. The other is the syringe barrel and a sheathed needle at one end and a coloured stopper on the other end (*Figure 6.4b*)
2. Remove the coloured stoppers from both component parts/tubes (do not

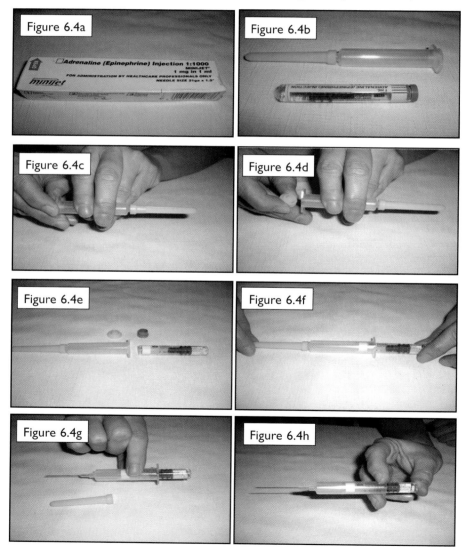

Figure 6.4a

Figure 6.4b

Figure 6.4c

Figure 6.4d

Figure 6.4e

Figure 6.4f

Figure 6.4g

Figure 6.4h

remove the needle sheathe at this stage as this will increase the likelihood of a needle-stick injury), one from the syringe barrel and one from the end of the glass drug tube (*Figures 6.4c* and *6.4d*)

3. The glass drug tube is then screwed into the top of the plastic syringe barrel (usually around 3 half turns) (*Figures 6.4e* and *6.4f*)
4. Depress the glass tube to expel the air out of the syringe and it is then ready for use (*Figures 6.4g* and *6.4h*).

Powder/liquid combinations: Drugs that are presented in this format are probably the most time consuming to prepare and draw up — the technique requires practice as mixing and transfer of the solution to a syringe is required. The presentation consists of a small bottle containing the powder and another small vial containing the liquid. Alternatively the liquid may sometimes be presented in a separate syringe containing a pre-measured quantity of liquid. The sequence of events for the pre-filled syringe is as follows:

1. Remove both items from the box (*Figure 6.5a* and *6.5b*)
2. Clean the bung in the top of the bottle with an alcohol wipe
3. Remove the needle cover and inject all the liquid into the bottle (*Figure 6.5c*)
4. Shake vigorously to ensure powder/liquid is mixed thoroughly and all the powder is dissolved
5. Draw the liquid back into the syringe (*Figure 6.5d*)
6. Administer the drug.

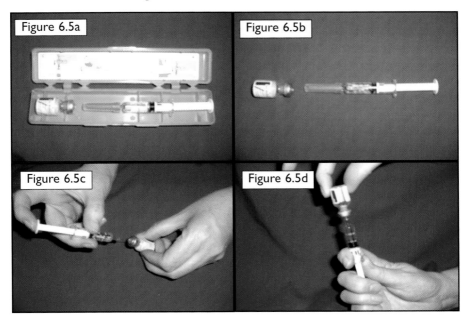

Ampoules: This is when the drug is supplied in a glass container with a narrowed neck. The top needs to be 'snapped' off and the drug is drawn to into a syringe ready to be injected. The liquid drug should be expelled from the top of the ampoule so that all the solution is available for drawing up, otherwise a significant proportion is lost when the ampoule is snapped open. A napkin or ampoule breaker should be used when breaking open the ampoule to avoid a sharps injury (*Figure 6.6*).

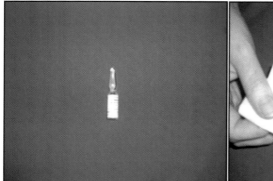 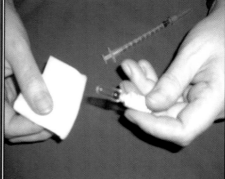

Figure 6.6a An ampoule.

Figure 6.6b Ready to 'snap' the top of the ampoule.

Alternative Routes

There are other methods of administering drugs that are used by paramedics and other trained personnel, but they would not be used by staff in a dental surgery and are included here for information only.

Intratracheal: It is possible for drugs to be absorbed via the trachea, but an endo-tracheal tube must have been inserted before using this route. Drugs, other than oxygen, cannot be administered via a laryngeal mask or any other type of airway aid. The drug is administered in a liquid form and injected directly down the endotracheal tube. Due to the variance in absorption rate the dose administered is usually double the dose used by other routes.

Intraosseous: This is used in paediatric resuscitation and involves using a trocar to insert a large bore rigid metal cannula into the medullary cavity of the tibia (shin) or sternum. Fluids can be administered through this route and drugs can be injected directly into the cannula and then 'flushed' through with fluid. The absorption rate is fairly rapid as the blood supply to the medullary bone spaces is profuse.

Emergency Drugs

Table 6.3 at the end of this chapter summarises the indications, routes of administration and dosages of the drugs mentioned below.

Oxygen

This should always be administered in an emergency situation; the only condition it will not help in is hyperventilation during a panic attack however it will not cause any harm. It should be administered directly to the patient using a facemask at a rate of not less than 5 litres per minute. However, when a patient is not breathing then the oxygen flow rate should be on maximum.

Glucose

This is used in the treatment of conscious hypoglycaemia and is administered orally. It is commercially available in the form of glucose powder which is mixed with water, or in proprietary gel preparations. Between 10-20g should be given. Alternative forms of glucose that can be given are glucose tablets, lozenges, sugar cubes (3 cubes is the equivalent of 10g of glucose), or 200 ml of milk. The glucose will be rapidly absorbed and elevate the blood sugars levels to a higher level.

Glucagon

This is used in the treatment of unconscious hypoglycaemia, and 1mg is administered by an IM injection. Glucagon is a hormone that is naturally produced by the pancreas and stimulates the conversion of glycogen into glucose, thus raising the circulating blood glucose levels. Its effects are quite short lasting so as soon as the patient becomes conscious oral glucose should be given to maintain a high blood glucose.

Aspirin

This is given to a patient who is suspected of having a myocardial infarction and is available as dispersible tablets in doses of 300mg. Aspirin has a direct action on the thrombotic potential of platelets by interference with the cyclo-oxygenase activity and thromboxane A2 synthesis; essentially it decreases platelet aggregation (i.e. their tendency to stick to one another), thus reducing clot formation.

Glyceryl trinitrate (GTN) spray

GTN spray is used to relieve the symptoms of angina. It is administered by spraying a metered dose directly under the tongue. Each actuation of the spray delivers 400µg of the drug, which is a potent vasodilator (causes the blood vessels to dilate). The nitrates in the spray are converted to nitric oxide which causes relaxation of the vascular smooth muscle, which has a more profound effect on the venous side of the circulation than the arterial side and thus reduces the load on the heart. In addition the nitrates have a direct dilatation effect on the coronary arteries thus increasing the blood flow to the heart muscle, and relieving the spasm. The side effects include flushing, headaches and a drop in blood pressure (due to the vasodilatation) but all of these are of short duration.

Salbutamol

Salbutamol is used for the emergency drug of asthma, and can also be used for severe bronchospasm during anaphylaxis. It is administered by inhalation using a metered dose of 100µg per actuation of an inhaler — usually two actuations are delivered — and it is administered every 10 minutes during an attack. In severe asthma attacks nebules of the drug (2.5-5.00mg) can be used in a nebuliser attached to an oxygen supply to produce a fine 'mist' which increases the delivered concentration. The drug is a selective short acting $beta_2$-adrenoreceptor agonist and works directly on the bronchial smooth muscle causing it to relax; this dilates the airway and reduces the resistance to air flow. Side effects can include a rapid heart rate and muscle tremors.

Midazolam

Benzodiazepines are used in the management of status epilepticus. Midazolam is now the treatment of choice in dental surgeries. Midazolam can be administered intravenously but the method of choice in a dental surgery setting is transmucosally. Midazolam, 10mg, can be administered by being deposited in the buccal sulcus using a syringe, or it can be administered intranasally using an atomisation device that attaches to the end of a syringe containing the required dose. The 10mg in 2ml preparation for injection can be given buccally or intranasally. There is a 10mg in 1ml buccal solution (Epistatus®) that can be placed in the buccal sulcus for transmucosal absorption.

Paramedics may carry diazepam for administration either rectally or intravenously. The rectal preparation is very often used in children and comes as a proprietary preparation with a measured dose contained in an applicator. The applicator is inserted and the dose delivered; it will then be absorbed transmucosally. The intravenous dose is 10mg, to be administered over 2 minutes, and the usual presentation is a glass ampoule containing 10mg of diazepam dissolved in 2mls of fluid.

Benzodiazepines produce a reduction in CNS activity by their interaction with benzodiazepine receptors, which facilitates the action of the inhibitory neurotransmitter gamma-aminobutyric acid. These drugs also cause respiratory depression and respiratory arrest can occur with overdose.

Adrenaline (Epinephrine)

This is the primary drug used in the treatment of anaphylaxis. It is administered by the IM route for anaphylaxis. The standard preparations contains 1mg of epinephrine in 1ml of fluid (1:1000 dilution) and this is administered in incremental doses of 0.5mg (0.5mls) every 5 minutes if necessary. Epinephrine is essential to help to reverse the respiratory and cardiovascular effects of acute allergic reactions. It is a powerful alpha-receptor agonist and causes peripheral vasoconstriction, thus stopping capillary leakage, maintaining circulatory volume and reducing oedema. It also has an effect on beta-receptors in the heart and lung. This causes relaxation of bronchial smooth muscle which dilates the airways and increases coronary blood flow and also the force of myocardial contraction so the circulation to the brain improves. Adrenaline also suppresses the release of histamine and leukotriene which are the chemical mediators responsible for the reaction.

There is another preparation of epinephrine, which some surgeries may carry, to be used in cardiac arrest. It has to be given intravenously (very difficult to do when the peripheral circulation has collapsed) and is a 1:10,000 dilution. 10mls are administered every 5 minutes during resuscitation attempts and then followed with a flush of fluid to ensure the drug is circulated.

Chlorphenamine

This is a second line treatment for anaphylaxis and can be administered by IV or IM routes, usually IM in a dental surgery setting. An adult dose is 10-20mg and it takes approximately 30 minutes to have any significant effect. It is an antihistamine and works as a histamine blocker, preventing further histamine release.

Hydrocortisone

This is used as a first line drug in the treatment of adrenal shock, and a second line drug in the treatment of anaphylaxis and status asthmaticus.

A single dose of 100-500mg is administered either IV or IM. If a patient with known adrenal suppression undergoes a steroid crisis then immediate elevation of the blood levels of hydrocortisone will reverse the effects. Hydrocortisone is a naturally produced glucocorticoid and it decreases the inflammatory process by suppressing the mediators of inflammation. It does take 4-6 hours to have an effect, which is why it is only considered as a second line treatment option for asthma and anaphylaxis.

Table 6.3   Summary of emergency drugs and their use in dental practice

Drug	Indication	Dose and Route of Administration
Oxygen	Most emergencies (not beneficial in hyperventilation)	Inhalation Supplemental oxygen - masks: 4-6 l/min - nasal cannula: 2-3 l/min Resuscitation - 10-15 l/min
Adrenaline (epinephrine)	Anaphylactic shock	0.5mg of 1:1000 (1mg/ml) repeated at 5 minute intervals if required >12 yrs: 500μg (0.5ml of 1:1000) 6-12yrs: 300μg (0.3ml of 1:1000) <6yrs: 150μg (0.15ml of 1:1000)
Glucose	Hypoglycaemia conscious patient	10-20g oral/buccal
Glucagon	Hypoglycaemia unconscious patient	1mg intramuscular, <8yrs: 500μg (0.5mg) intramuscular
Salbutamol	Asthma	200μg (2xpuffs) inhalation
Glyceryl trinitrate	Cardiac chest pain/ angina	400μg metered dose sublingual
Aspirin	Myocardial infarct	300mg oral

continued....

Midazolam	*Status epilepticus*	10mg buccal or intranasal (child dose: transmucosal midazolam 200µg/kg) 1-5yrs: 5mg 5-10yrs: 7.5mg >10yrs: 10mg
Chlorphenamine*	Anaphylaxis 2nd line drug	10-20mg intramuscular or slow intravenous. For doses in children see chapter 8
Hydrocortisone*	Anaphylaxis 2nd line drug *status asthmaticus* 2nd line drug adrenal shock 1st line drug	100-500mg intravenous or intramuscular. For doses in children see chapter 8

*The BNF removed both chlorphenamine and hydrocortisone from their recommended list of emergency drugs for dental practice

CHAPTER 7

Assessment of the Sick Patient

When a person starts to feel unwell the initial symptoms they are complaining about often tend to be vague and non-specific. At this stage it can be impossible for a healthcare professional to make a definitive diagnosis as to the cause of the problem, and certainly it is not possible to instigate any definitive treatment. Members of the dental team are not comfortable with events that are outside of their control; they are used to understanding their patients' dental needs and providing planned care. Dental staff like to act on information received or deduced from a situation and react accordingly. In a medical emergency, however, this information may be difficult to obtain. Patients are often non-specific about their symptoms, and many of the initial presenting symptoms for medical emergencies are similar. When a patient becomes pale, sweaty and feels unwell it could be a simple faint, hypoglycaemia or the beginning of anaphylactic shock. A method is, therefore, needed to systematically obtain the necessary information and act upon it in a rational manner. A systematic approach will help give structure and purpose to the management of the situation and this will reassure the team, the patient and any relatives who may be present. The method proposed will also allow the severity of the situation to be assessed, monitored and the success of any interventions verified.

It is not necessary to have a definitive diagnosis when managing an emergency, as there are fundamental principles that apply to all emergency situations, and a methodical analysis of the patient's signs and symptoms will ensure that the healthcare professional feels that they have 'done all they can' to the best of their ability. This method of assessment is used universally by all emergency healthcare personnel and is called the A,B,C,D,E approach:

- **A** is airway
- **B** is breathing
- **C** is circulation
- **D** is disability
- **E** is exposure.

It does not matter whether the patient is conscious or unconscious, the assessment is the same. It is always carried out in this order, and any problems identified are dealt with before progressing to the next stage of the assessment. Anything that you do during the course of the assessment is called 'an intervention', for example clearing an airway. The assessment is repeated each time you do an intervention, or if anything about the patient's condition changes, such as losing or regaining consciousness. Each stage of the assessment is described below.

Airway

The dental team need to establish if the patient has an open (or patent) airway. Is there any sign of airway blockage such as the presence of fluids or vomit? If the patient is unconscious is the tongue blocking the airway? Carry out appropriate interventions to open the airway such as removing debris with a finger-sweep, or suction or improving the airway with a jaw thrust. Once the airway has been assessed and any intervention undertaken proceed to assessing the patient's breathing.

Breathing

Is the patient breathing and if so how effective is it? Breathing is assessed as described earlier in the book. If the patient is not breathing, then follow the basic life support (BLS) algorithm in calling for assistance and undertake artificial ventilations. If the patient is breathing spontaneously then it needs to be assessed for how efficacious it is. This will give you more information about the patients condition and give insight into whether the primary problem is a respiratory cause. The following need to be considered:

- Is there any noise associated with the respiration?
- What type of noise is it and is it occurring on inspiration or expiration?
- What is the respiratory rate? If 8 breaths per minute or below then additional ventilations must be supplied. A rate of 12 to 20 is acceptable. Above this rate there may be insufficient oxygen being absorbed.
- Is the patient using accessory muscles to draw in the air?
- Is the chest expansion equal and are both sides of the chest inflating?
- A pulse oximeter, if available, is a useful piece of equipment as it will tell you the arterial oxygen saturation.

Following this you may decide to administer high flow oxygen. After this has been done breathing should be re-assessed to see the effect it has had on the patient. Ensure the patient is in the most comfortable and appropriate position. A conscious patient with a respiratory problem often wants to sit upright and slightly forward. An unconscious patient with spontaneous respiration should be placed in the recovery position if possible.

Circulation

Does the patient have a reasonable circulation? The circulation should be checked and if there is no central pulse you should commence cardiopulmonary resuscitation (CPR) immediately. If there is evidence of a circulation then the following parameters need to be assessed:

- The quality of the pulse. A patient's pulse should be taken both centrally and peripherally and needs to be measured over a minimum of 10 seconds. The features to look for are the rate, is the rate regular or irregular and the volume of the pulse both centrally and peripherally and any differences between them
- The patient's skin colour — is it pale or normal?
- Does the skin feel warm or cold?
- Blood pressure should be measured and recorded
- Capillary Refill Time (CRT).

If a patient is going into shock their peripheral circulation begins to close down in an effort to centralise the circulating blood volume and maintain the blood supply to the heart and brain. The capillaries in the limbs shut down quite early during this process, so another good measure of what is happening is to apply cutaneous pressure for five seconds on a fingertip held at heart level, or just above, with sufficient pressure to cause blanching. Time how long it takes for the skin colour to return to normal when the pressure is released. This is called the capillary refill time (CRT). A normal CRT for this would be 2 seconds, although cold surroundings and age can increase this slightly. A prolonged CRT is an indicator of reduced peripheral perfusion.

The only active intervention to influence circulation that can be easily done in a dental surgery is to change the patient's position. This is an attempt to encourage the blood in the limbs to be redistributed into the central circulation. If a patient is put in the supine position the effect of this intervention should be reassessed. It should be remembered that laying a patient flat is not always helpful — it can adversely increase the load on the heart and also cause breathing difficulties.

Disability

The patient's level of consciousness is assessed using the AVPU scale (alert/verbal/painful/unresponsive), this is an assessment of the central nervous system (CNS). The patient's pupil reaction is measured by using the dental light. When the CNS is depressed the patient requires transfer to a hospital as soon as possible. If there is a glucose monitor available then it is worth measuring blood glucose. One very simple intervention is to administer glucose if the level is low.

Exposure

It is helpful to briefly examine the patient's skin on the face, arms and legs for any rashes and ankles for oedema. In a medical emergency the peripheral circulation usually 'shuts down', and the unwell patient should therefore be kept warm to reduce heat loss, and this can easily be achieved by producing a blanket.

It is good practice to write down all the findings during the assessment as this provides good documentation for transfer to paramedics should this be necessary. *Table 7.1* summarises the A,B,C,D,E assessment.

Table 7.1   Summary of the A,B,C,D assessment

Assessment	Parameters	Interventions
Airway	Patent, open, clear	Head tilt-chin lift, jaw thrust, suction, oropharyngeal or nasopharyngeal airways, oxygen
Breathing	Rate, depth, accessory muscles, bilateral	Oxygen, chair position, drugs as applicable. Consider salbutamol if expiratory wheeze
Circulation	Pulse rate, volume, central versus peripheral, blood pressure, capillary refill time	Position chair, drugs as applicable
Disability	alert/verbal/painful/ unresponsive scale, eye pupils, blood, glucose	Position, glucose (possible glucagon if patient is unconscious and has low blood glucose)
Exposure	Rashes, ankle oedema, heat loss	Keep warm with a blanket

Scenario

The use of this systematic assessment method will help in the diagnosis of the primary problem and thus enable a treatment decision to be taken. It is not necessary to identify what has caused the emergency, merely to compensate for the effects the problem is causing. *Box 7.1* overleaf is a worked example to illustrate this point and show how useful the assessment process is.

Box 7.1: Case Study

A 70-year-old woman is attending the practice for a restoration on a lower first molar. This woman is a regular patient at the practice and is healthy. She has no relevant medical history, and does not take any medication. Despite being a regular attendee she is nervous when having treatment. Just after the administration of the ID block she becomes pale and sweaty and states that she 'feels awful'.

The initial thoughts here on a possible cause for her signs and symptoms include a potential faint, a panic attack, intravascular injection of local anaesthetic, or some other but unknown cause. Hopefully by carrying out a systematic assessment the cause may be identified. The results of the A,B,C,D,E assessment is as described below.

Airway: The patient is talking without distress and is not choking so therefore her airway is currently clear.

Breathing: The patient is breathing quickly with a respiration rate of 40 breaths per minute, leaning forward and she is using her accessory muscles of respiration. Her chest expansion is equal but there is no noise associated with her breathing.
The breathing rate is faster than it should be. The dental team need to decide if an intervention is necessary. The patient is sitting forward — this is a comfortable position for her and it does not need to be altered. The patient may be hyperventilating due to panic, in which case we could ask her re-breathe from cupped hands or a paper bag. Alternatively, she may have insufficient oxygen in which case it would be sensible to administer additional high flow oxygen. Decide on one course of action and re-assess to determine if the intervention was successful or had an adverse effect on the patient's condition.
Re-breathing increases her respiration rate, so this intervention is stopped. The patient is given high-flow oxygen and the reassessment shows an improvement in her breathing rate, which slows down to 25 breaths per minute. Oxygen is therefore a good intervention and also excludes the diagnosis of hyperventilation (oxygen would not normally improve hyperventilation).

Circulation: The patient's pulse rate is 145 beats per minute and irregular. This is cause for concern as she has a fast and irregular heart rate. The capillary refill time is 5 seconds, indicating some peripheral shutdown, and her blood pressure is 170/90 mmHg. This patient's blood pressure is a good sign as she is maintaining her circulation at the moment.

Disability: The patient remains at A (alert) on the AVPU scale; her pupils reaction to light is normal and her blood glucose is 4; within normal range

Exposure: The patient is provided with a blanket and there is no obvious rash or ankle oedema.

At this stage we know that she has two physiological systems affected: respiratory and cardiac. These systems are interrelated but it would be helpful to work out where the primary problem has occurred. The patient's respiratory rate decreased with oxygen, but a key piece of information was that her respiration was not noisy — there is no indication of obstruction such as a wheeze. It is therefore unlikely that the origin of the problem is primarily respiratory. The irregular pulse rate implies that something has occurred in the heart, but the blood pressure reassures us that it is not catastrophic at this stage. In a dental surgery setting there is no further interventions that the team can do, other than arrange her transfer to hospital as she is not well enough to go home.

The assessment has allowed the dental team to make decisions and take actions using a rational and controlled approach. This is reassuring for both the staff and the patient.

Do you know what the diagnosis is?

Answer: Atrial fibrillation

Section 3

Medical Emergencies

CHAPTER 8

Anaphylaxis

DEFINITION

Anaphylaxis, also known as anaphylactic shock or anaphylactic crisis, is a severe allergic reaction that is a serious and potentially life threatening condition that can result in respiratory and/or circulatory collapse. Immediate medical management is required

PREDISPOSING FACTORS

Atopic individual

Exposure to allergens (triggers)

SIGNS AND SYMPTOMS

- Flushing (erythema) of the skin
- Abdominal pain, vomiting, diarrhoea
- Itching
- Weak rapid pulse
- Hypotension (profound drop in blood pressure)
- Loss of consciousness
- Altered sensations, numbness and tingling of hands and feet
- Skin rash
- Oedema of face and airways
- Stridor and wheezing

MANAGEMENT

- Call for assistance from other surgery staff
- Call for paramedics
- Consider adjusting chair position[1]:
    flat if patient has low blood pressure or is unconscious
    patient with breathing problems may prefer to be upright
- Give oxygen
- Prepare 1:1000 adrenaline for administration of 0.5ml (0.5mg) injection intramuscularly every 5 minutes
- Continue to monitor patient (ABCDE)
- Consider giving salbutamol inhaler if symptoms are mainly respiratory
- Consider preparing the second line drugs for administration[2]:
    chlorphenamine 10-20mg intramuscular or subcutaneous
    hydrocortisone 100-500mg intravenous

PAEDIATRIC DOSES

Adrenaline — intramuscular injection

> 12 years: 500µg (0.5ml of 1:1000)

6–12 years: 300µg (0.3ml of 1:1000)

< 6 years: 150µg (0.15ml of 1:1000)

[1] Note effect of the intervention

[2] Some practices may not have these two drugs as they are not required for first line management. For second line drugs (chlorphenamine and hydrocortisone) please see text

Anaphylaxis is a potentially fatal allergic reaction. The allergic reaction (also known as a hypersensitivity response) may develop slowly, or can occur very quickly depending upon how the patient was exposed to the allergic substance, the route of administration, and their individual response. Examples of the allergy triggering substance — an allergen — includes food products, drugs, latex or insect stings. Perhaps the most well known are peanut allergy or an allergy to the penicillins. In dentistry, possible allergens are natural rubber latex and drugs such as penicillins or non-steroidal anti-inflammatory drugs (for example ibuprofen). The injectable local anaesthetic agents used today are highly unlikely to cause an allergic reaction. However, some topical local anaesthetics (the ester containing agents) such as amethocaine (tetracaine) and benzocaine can cause allergic reactions; fortunately these tend to be less severe Type IV (delayed hypersensitivity) reactions rather than an anaphylaxis. Patients often say they are allergic to a substance when in fact they mean they have experienced a side-effect to a medicine or the medicine made them feel unwell in some way.

Physiological Explanation

The immune system is part of the body's defence system against harmful substances such as bacteria. One of the ways that it does this is by recognising 'foreign' proteins — such as those found on the surface of viruses and bacteria. Some of the white blood cells, lymphocytes, recognise these proteins as foreign and produce antibodies which can neutralise, or inactivate the protein preventing it from causing any bodily damage. There are different types of lymphocytes; some (the plasma cells) produce the antibody, and others have a memory which 'remember' the individual foreign protein once it has been sensitised (exposed to the antigen). When the body mounts an allergic response it can do so in varying ways. Two types of allergic response — Type I and Type IV — are of relevance to dentistry:

- The Type IV allergy is a delayed hypersensitivity response and is often seen as skin rashes. This can be uncomfortable and distressing but is not life-threatening and is not relevant to anaphylaxis. An example of a Type IV response that is frequently seen is the skin reaction that develops to inexpensive costume jewellery. Another example is seen in dental staff who develop an allergic contact dermatitis to some of the chemicals present in latex gloves. Type IV allergic reactions occur more commonly than Type I reactions.

- Type I reactions have the potential to be life threatening.

During a Type I hypersensitivity response the immune cells release various natural chemicals, one of which is histamine. Histamine causes dilation of the blood vessels and also causes the walls of the vessel to become 'leaky' to fluids so that the area affected becomes swollen and oedematous, thus diluting the antigen. Cell bound IgE is present in higher concentrations in the bronchial tree, the dermis, the gastro-intestinal tract and the mucosa in the nose so these are the areas predominantly affected by a repeat exposure to the allergen, for example as in hayfever where exposure to pollen produces sneezing, red rashes on the skin if it has come into contact with it, and wheezing.

If a patient who has had a previous exposure to an allergen and has been sensitised to it, suffers a repeat exposure, there is an overproduction of the IgE that results in a massive release of histamine which effectively makes the whole circulatory system leaky to water, the water passes out of the bloodstream and into the tissues. This obviously reduces the effective blood volume which produces the drop in blood pressure, the blood content becomes thick and sluggish due to the lack of water, and the tissue spaces fill up with fluid, which is why there is obvious swelling, particularly of the airways and face because there is a concentration of cell bound IgE in these areas. The swelling causes potential airway blockage and the lungs effectively begin to fill with water reducing the oxygen exchange available.

Although the theoretical ideal treatment would appear to be administration of an 'antihistamine' to reverse the histamine effects this is actually too slow, and the initial treatment is to stop and hopefully reverse the capillary dilatation and water leakage. This is why it is essential to administer adrenaline because this causes immediate vasoconstriction and 'closes' the blood vessels down very quickly. High flow oxygen is also a priority as this helps to increase the inspired concentration to compensate for the lungs inefficiency. The other essential is to raise the blood pressure which in a dental surgery setting can only be done by lying the patient flat and elevating the legs, and care needs to be taken if the patient is struggling to breathe.

In a hospital setting, or when the paramedics arrive, administration of intra-venous fluid is a priority as this replaces the fluid lost into the tissues and restores the blood pressure rapidly. The administration of an antihistamine and a steroid also helps to reduce the inflammatory response but they are a 'second line' treatment.

Signs and Symptoms

A casualty may show some or all of the following signs and symptoms:

- Flushing (erythema) of the skin

- Abdominal pain, vomiting and diarrhoea
- Itching
- Weak rapid pulse
- Hypotension (profound drop in blood pressure)
- Loss of consciousness
- Altered sensations, numbness and tingling of the hands and feet
- Skin rash
- Oedema of face and airways
- Stridor and wheezing.

Essentially an anaphylactic reaction will result in one or both of the following:

- A profound drop in blood pressure
- Respiratory distress.

Both the respiratory difficulty and the circulatory collapse can result in loss of consciousness and, if untreated, death. If there is any suspicion that a patient might be beginning to suffer from this condition the paramedics should be called immediately as the patient may deteriorate rapidly. The dental team have a valuable role to play in trying to improve the patient's condition before the arrival of the emergency services.

The signs and symptoms alerting staff to the onset of anaphylaxis can vary tremendously and include facial flushing, altered sensations sometimes described as 'pins and needles' may occur. Signs of allergy can be apparent by an itching of the skin, a skin rash and the appearance of small 'heat spots' or hives on the skin. Facial swelling — oedema — can develop and can be pronounced orally involving the lips and tongue. Oropharyngeal oedema may occur and cause respiratory distress. Breathing problems can also occur from bronchospasm. Patients who have experienced anaphylaxis often describe it as 'an impending sense of doom'.

Management

Expert help is required to manage anaphylaxis. The immediate or emergency treatment of anaphylaxis involves the administration of adrenaline as soon as possible. This consists of giving 0.5mg of adrenaline intramuscularly, this is 0.5ml of 1 in 1000 (0.5mg is equal to 500µg). High flow oxygen is also essential to help ensure adequate oxygenation, as gas exchange in the lungs may be impaired.

The casualty should be placed in a comfortable position. Ideally the blood pressure should be raised by lying the patient flat and elevating the legs. If the patient is unconscious this is not a problem, however, care needs to be taken if the patient is struggling to breathe. When patients have respiratory distress they prefer to sit upright or forward.

If the tongue is swelling and the patient is unconscious then an oropharyngeal airway may be advisable, alternatively a nasopharyngeal airway may be used.

The administration of an antihistamine and a steroid are given to help stabilise the patient's condition. These drugs do not work immediately but contribute to long-term stability of the patient. These drugs constitute 'second line' treatment and not essential in a dental surgery setting.

To help restore or maintain the casualties blood pressure administration of intra-venous fluid is a priority as this replaces the fluid lost from the circulation. The paramedics will put a drip up as a matter of priority.

Care has to be exercised with doses of drugs for children; they need to be appropriately reduced. The paediatric doses of adrenaline and the second-line drugs chlorphenamine and hydrocortisone are also given for completion in *Table 8.1*.

Prevention

Allergies affect about 10% of the population, which means that roughly 1 in 10 patients will give a positive history. It is no surprise therefore that every patient

Table 8.1   Paediatric drug regimes in anaphylaxis

Drug	Dose	Route
Adrenaline		Intramuscular
> 12 years	500µg (0.5ml of 1:1000)	
6–12 years	300µg (0.3ml of 1:1000)	
< 6 years	0.15µg (0.15ml of 1:1000)	
Chlorphenamine		Intramuscular
> 12 years	10mg	or slow intravenous
6–12 years	5mg	
< 6 months–6 years	2.5mg	
Hydrocortisone		Intramuscular
> 12 years	200mg	or slow intravenous
6–12 years	100mg	
< 6 months–6 years	50mg	

should always be questioned carefully about any history of possible allergic reactions and any known allergen must be avoided. When a patient has a history of atopy (childhood eczema and allergic asthma) they have a tendency to develop allergies, and staff should be alert to this. Many patients will, on a seasonal basis, be taking antihistamines for pollen allergies to minimise their symptoms. However, patients who are considered to be at a significant risk of developing anaphylaxis will very often carry an Epipen®, which contains 300μg of adrenaline, for self-administration. The individual will have received training in how to use the self-injector should they begin to feel the symptoms of anaphylaxis developing.

There are certain allergens that are associated with producing anaphylaxis and some of these are very relevant to dental treatment, and include penicillins, cephalosporins, natural rubber latex (NRL), aspirin, and intra-venous general anaesthetic agents. Food allergies are often important because there are associations between certain allergies to fruits and nuts that are associated with NRL. Foods reported as having cross-sensitivity with NRL include chestnuts, kiwi fruit and bananas. If a patient gives any history of atopy and has multiple allergies it is advisable to be extremely cautious when prescribing medications, especially when using new drugs that have only recently become available. It is also worth remembering that some of the newer haemostatic agents are produced from shellfish, which is a common food allergy.

As NRL is a well-known allergen it is best practice to avoid purchasing items of dental equipment that are known to contain NRL when NRL-free alternatives are readily available. The use of NRL gloves in NHS hospitals has been stopped and they now exclusively use NRL-free gloves.

When there is uncertainty around the true nature of an allergy reported by a patient further information or advice should be sought. If a patients medical practitioner is uncertain as to the patient's allergy history regarding a product that a dentist is likely to use then the patient may need to be referred to an allergist or immunologist for further testing.

CHAPTER 9

Angina and Myocardial Infarction

DEFINITIONS Angina	Myocardial Infarction (MI)
Pain or discomfort in the chest due to reduced blood flow and oxygen in the heart	Damage or death to an area of the heart muscle resulting from reduced or blocked blood supply. A myocardial infarction is also called a coronary thrombosis or heart attack)
PREDISPOSING FACTORS • History of coronary heart disease • High blood cholesterol • Age (middle age or older) • Patients who have risk factors for coronary artery disease (e.g. diabetes, obesity, hypertension, family history of coronary heart disease)	As for angina but also: • Previous history of MI • Recent history of an MI (especially within the first 12 weeks of recovery)
SIGNS AND SYMPTOMS • Crushing feeling of a weight bearing down on the chest more or less • Central chest pain • Breathlessness • Sweating • Fear • Regular fast pulse	• Severe chest pain which may radiate to the left arm or jaw • Shortness of breath • Weakness • Fatigue • Pallor • Sweating • Anxiety • Nausea • Irregular pulse and palpitations
MANAGEMENT • GTN spray • Oxygen • Sitting upright • Reassurance • Monitor ABC • Note time when symptoms started • If pain continues assume patient is having an MI and call for paramedics	• High flow oxygen • GTN spray • Aspirin 300mg • Call paramedics • Nitrous oxide if available • Monitor ABC • Note time when symptoms started • Transfer to paramedics

This chapter covers two cardiac emergencies, angina and myocardial infarction. It is logical that they are covered together because both are the result of coronary artery disease and share common risk factors, management strategies, and the population cohort is similar. Myocardial infarction is the leading cause of death worldwide. Coronary heart disease is the leading cause of death in the UK. It affects men more than women, but the chances of having the disease increases with age. There are currently around 1.2 million people in the UK who suffer from angina (about 1 in 50 people), with one in every four men, and one in every six women dying from the disease. In the UK, approximately 300,000 people have a heart attack each year. The risk factors associated with developing coronary artery disease are listed in *Table 9.1*.

Table 9.1   Risk factors associated with coronary artery disease

Increasing age (middle age and older)	Excessive alcohol consumption
Obesity	Disorders of lipid metabolism
Hypertension	Hypercholesterolaemia
Smoking	Chronic stress
Family history	Drug abuse
Diabetes	Lack of exercise

Physiology

Coronary artery disease

The blood supply to the heart muscle — the myocardium — is provided by the right and left coronary arteries; these are the first vessels to branch off the aorta. *Figure 9.1* shows this. The structure of these arteries is similar to other arteries and consists of a muscular outer layer and a thin lining layer (the endothelium) on the inside. Fat can deposit on this inside layer forming a series of waxy lipid patches called plaques or atheromatous plaques (atherosclerosis or arteriosclerosis). These plaques cause the inside surface of the arteries to become roughened and further deposition of plaque increases the thickness of the atheromatous plaques. The lumen of the vessel begins to dramatically narrow and this significantly reduces the blood flow to the heart muscle. This is demonstrated in *Figures 9.2a-c*.

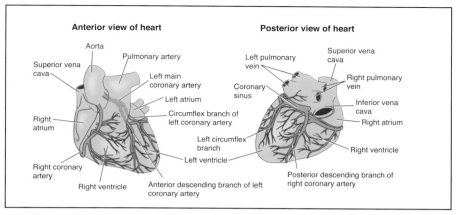

Figure 9.1 The coronary arteries which supply blood to the heart

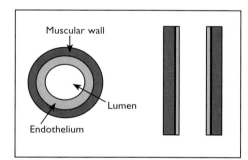

Figure 9.2a Healthy vessel

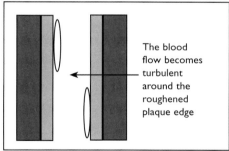

Figure 9.2b Irregular fatty plaques begin to form

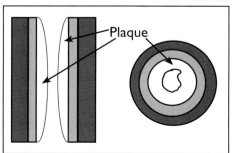

Figure 9.2c The lumen of the vessel becomes progressively narrower as the layers build up

Angina

Angina is the name for the medical signs and symptoms that result from the narrowed coronary arteries. When a person is resting the heart is beating at its resting rate; when any type of exertion is undertaken the heart is required to beat more strongly and at a faster rate to ensure an adequate supply of oxygenated blood is being circulated to the active tissues. The more strenuous the exertion, the more cardiac effort is required, and the more oxygen the heart will need.

When the coronary arteries are narrowed less blood is being supplied directly to the heart muscle, so a situation will be reached where the demand of the heart muscle for blood will exceed that which the coronary arteries can supply. The heart muscle will therefore become deprived of oxygen and effectively suffers from 'cramps', producing severe pain. This type of pain is called 'ischaemic' pain — meaning 'deprived of blood and oxygen'. The level of activity that produces the pain is an indication of the degree of occlusion of the arteries. When pain only occurs on strenuous exercise then there is still quite a good blood supply. When the pain is occurring on very minor exertion, e.g. walking a short distance, then this is an indication of a severe narrowing of the coronary arteries and the patient will be advised to have a surgery, such as the placement of stents (to open the coronary vessels) or even a coronary artery bypass graft (CABG) to restore adequate cardiac circulation.

There are three types of angina. With **stable angina** the pain is brought on by exertion and lasts only a few minutes if the activity is stopped. The heartbeat remains regular throughout the attack. Most patients who have this type of angina will carry antiangina medication to use when the pain occurs (such as glyceryl trinitrate). A patient who has stable angina may well progress to having **unstable angina** if the coronary artery disease progresses causing a further narrowing of the arteries. In this form the pain is produced by very little effort, and may even occur at rest. Patients who have this form of angina have a significant risk of having a myocardial infarction. In **variant angina** the attacks are not related to coronary artery disease and the pain is caused by the coronary arteries suddenly going into spasm and narrowing. When a patient who suffers from this has an attack it can be associated with cardiac conduction problems and the heartbeat can become very irregular.

Signs and symptoms

The symptoms of angina can be variable depending upon the severity of the coronary disease. It can be a mild, uncomfortable feeling that is similar to indigestion. A severe angina attack, however, can cause a feeling of heaviness, or tightness, usually in the centre of the chest, which may radiate to the left arm and jaw. The chest pain may be likened to a heavy weight pressing on the chest. Respiratory symptoms also develop, usually the patient is breathing very quickly and begins to pant, they may complain that they cannot breathe; there is also a very strong feeling of fear. Angina is often triggered by physical activity or emotionally stressful situations. The symptoms usually pass within about 10-15 minutes and can be relieved by resting or using a nitrate tablet or spray. If the symptoms persist the diagnosis should be reconsidered as it is likely that the patient is having a myocardial infarction.

Management

Patients often want to sit upright and lean slightly forward as this makes it easier to breathe so this position should be encouraged. Under no circumstances insist that the patient lies flat. High flow oxygen should be administered and the patient should be helped to use their rescue medication — usually one spray of GTN sublingually. This rescue medication works by causing the muscle in the walls of the coronary arteries to dilate thus widening the effective size of the lumen of the blood vessel which in turn increases the blood flow. A further dose can be administered if the first is ineffective.

If the pain does not reduce, and continues for 15 minutes with no sign of abating despite the GTN, then a myocardial infarction should be suspected and the patient transferred to hospital. A patient who has angina is familiar with their own condition and will tell you what is 'normal' for them during an attack, if they say that this is worse than normal, or less responsive than normal, then immediate transfer to hospital is required.

Many more people could recover from heart attacks if they got help faster. Of the people who die from heart attacks about half die within an hour of the first symptoms and before they reach the hospital.

Myocardial Infarction

A myocardial infarction (MI) is the medical term for a heart attack. It is caused by a complete occlusion of one of the coronary arteries, which results in the area of myocardium supplied by that vessel being completely deprived of its blood supply and therefore this area of muscle will die. The usual cause of this is either for a clot (a thrombus) to form on the roughened surface of wall of the blood vessel or for a plaque to rupture and causes a blockage. In either event the blood flow stops at the blockage because the clot completely occludes the lumen of the vessel. Obviously the severity of the infarction will determine the outcome, if the clot occurs in a vessel supplying a large area of muscle then the heart is unlikely to be able to continue to beat and a cardiac arrest will result, if the area supplied is relatively small then it may be possible for the rest of the cardiac muscle to compensate and normal cardiac function can be re-established. Depending upon the size of the problem the patient may or may not experience pain.

Signs and symptoms

These are caused by the death of the area of heart muscle, and the resulting effects on the body described as 'cardiogenic' shock — a shock of cardiac origin. The signs and symptoms are variable and it is important to remember that 30% of heart attacks are **silent** as they do not produce any obvious symptoms, although fatigue usually occurs. In contrast, a massive heart attack can quickly result in a cardiac arrest. A heart attack can happen at any time, including during rest. The classic symptom is chest discomfort and pain and is similar to that of angina, but it is often more severe. Unlike angina, the symptoms of an MI cannot be relieved using a nitrate tablet or spray. If the symptoms last longer than 15 minutes, it is probably a heart attack. During a heart attack the following clinical features may also be seen:

- A feeling of heaviness in the chest
- Pain resembling indigestion (heartburn)
- Sweating
- Light-headedness
- Nausea
- Breathlessness
- Cardiac arrest.

Management

Early recognition is very important because the patient needs to be transferred to a coronary care unit as soon as possible. The initial infarct may be minor, but because there is an increased load on the rest of the cardiac muscle, a second catastrophic infarct can follow within 24 hours.

The primary aim of treatment is supportive, there is an acronym used for the treatment of an MI called MONA — Morphine, Oxygen, Nitrate and Aspirin. Three of these can be administered in a dental surgery. If a patient has a history of angina and used GTN spray then it is worth administering this as it will dilate the arteries and may help to relieve some of the symptoms, if they have never used GTN then it is unwise to administer this without cardiac monitoring as it will cause the patient to drop their blood pressure. High flow oxygen should be administered together with aspirin which will help to prevent further clot formation. Most dental surgeries do not carry morphine, but nitrous oxide can be administered (as long as the oxygen concentration is maintained) as this will help to provide some pain relief.

The patient should be positioned so that their legs are straight (to prevent excess cardiac loading by venous return) and their back is at 45 degrees as this aids breathing, if a patient wishes to sit forwards they should be allowed to do so. If a patient is conscious they should not be positioned flat as this will increase cardiac load. If they become unconscious they will have to be placed in the recovery position to allow airway control. Patients need to be constantly reassured and monitored for ABC and care should be taken as vomiting is common and may cause airway obstruction. The paramedics will apply cardiac monitoring leads on arrival and may well administer streptokinase immediately. This type of drug is colloquially called a 'clotbuster' and there is good evidence to suggest that early administration of these drugs can help the long-term prognosis, however they are only suitable for certain types of infarct.

Prevention of Cardiac Emergencies

A thorough medical history should alert the clinician to any risk factors.

Patients who have angina will normally carry their rescue medication in the form of a GTN spray. This should always be placed in an accessible area when a patient is having treatment. If they do not have their own medication with them then the surgery's GTN spray from the emergency drug box should be readily available.

It is also sensible to ensure that patients who suffers from angina should not have to exert themselves. If they have rushed to the appointment they should be given time to rest before treatment. Patients with unstable angina may not be able to climb the stairs to reach surgeries that are on the first floor. It is a good idea to ask a patient with coronary heart disease, just before any treatment, if it is problematic. It is unwise to treat such a patient if they are felling unwell.

Stressful situations cause cardiac exertion in a similar way to exercise, so it is important to reduce any stress caused by dental pain or fear as these can precipitate an angina attack. If the patient suffers from dental anxiety then it may be prudent to consider sedation for any treatment that the patient perceives to be stressful; this may need to be undertaken in a hospital environment or specialist clinic and will be dependent upon the severity of the coronary heart disease.

When a patient gives a recent history of an MI it is wise to delay elective treatment. This is because the myocardium is unstable following an infarction and dental treatment can precipitate abnormal heart rhythms (arrhythmias) and further infarctions. The time period when it is safe to commence treatment cannot accurately be specified and will vary for different patients and dental procedures. The main risk is in the first 6 weeks post-MI. Some textbooks advise no elective treatment for 6 months, but this time delay may be over cautious and is based on morbidity and mortality statistics from general surgery carried out under general anaesthesia. Certainly, the risks are higher for surgery and general anaesthesia than for routine restorative procedures. It is therefore necessary to assess a patient's suitability for dental treatment individually.

CHAPTER 10

Asthma

DEFINITION	
An asthma attack consists of widespread narrowing of the bronchial airways	
PREDISPOSING FACTORS	
• Exposure to triggers/antigens	
• Stress	
• Poorly controlled asthma	
• Concurrent infection or illness	
SIGNS AND SYMPTOMS	
• Coughing	
• Expiratory Wheezing	
• Difficulty in breathing	
• Anxiety and distress	
• Using accessory muscles to breathe	
• Cyanosis	
MANAGEMENT	
• Administer bronchodilators — use patient's own 'reliever' inhaler or of necessary use the surgery inhaler which is usually salbutamol. Administer 2 puffs (100µg per actuation)	
• Repeat if ineffective but use a spacer device, if available, or use a nebuliser, if available, to administer 2.5-5mg salbutamol	
• Phone paramedics if no improvement	
• Administer oxygen	
• Ensure patient is in a comfortable position and reassure	
• Monitor ABC	
PAEDIATRIC DRUG DOSES	
Children's drug doses as above	

Asthma is a very common medical condition, with approximately 5.2 million sufferers in the UK. The dental team must not become complacent with this common condition, however, as it is also a potentially life threatening condition with up to 1,200 deaths being recorded annually as being due to asthma or asthma-related conditions. Asthma occurs when the small airways — the bronchi and bronchioles — become narrow and make breathing difficult and laboured. The patient will cough and wheeze on expiration. The narrowing, or constriction, of the bronchial airways occurs as a result of being exposed to an asthma trigger. If the attack is protracted and uncontrolled the patient will be struggling to breathe, become severely distressed, develop a rapid heartbeat and may begin to turn blue from cyanosis. As mentioned previously death can occur if expert help is obtained too late.

Physiology

For inhaled oxygen to reach the alveoli of the lungs, it has to pass through the bronchi and bronchioles of the lower airways. The space available for the air to pass in and out of these airways is dependent upon how patent the lumen of these tubes are — how large the diameter is. The wider this tube is, the less resistance there is to air movement, so breathing should be effortless, and a maximum volume of air can pass in and out of the lungs with each breath.

The bronchi and bronchioles are effectively composed of three parts, a circular ring of muscle, a layer of ciliated lining cells, and a thin coating of mucous produced by the lining cells (*Figure 10.1*). Problems with the transport of oxygen in and out of the lungs occur if there is a reduction in the patency of the lower airway and any of the three layers of tissue can reduce the size, or patency, of the airway. If the smooth muscle in the tubular walls contracts this will reduce the diameter. If the cell layer lining the walls becomes inflamed

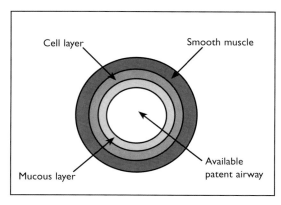

Cell layer

Smooth muscle

Mucous layer

Available patent airway

Figure 10.1 Cross-section of the lower bronchial airways.

then fluid will build up below the surface narrowing the diameter, and if the mucous layer becomes thicker this will narrow the lumen of the airway.

In asthma an exposure to a triggering agent will produce a marked contraction of the smooth muscle, a severe irritation in the lining cells causing them to swell up, and an excessive production of thick adherent mucous will obstruct the walls of the lumen. The effective diameter, or patency, of the airway becomes narrowed and compromises the movement of air. Considerable effort is required to generate sufficient pressure to actually allow breathing, which is difficult. The air is forced out against the narrowed airways and produces the characteristic expiratory wheezing sound. The more pronounced and audible the wheeze, the narrower the airways have become. The respiratory effort becomes progressively more difficult which produces stress, which exacerbates the situation, and the situation steadily worsens. If the attack is prolonged this is called 'status asthmaticus' and the patient becomes exhausted with the respiratory effort and may die.

Symptoms and Signs

Acute asthma, or an asthma attack, is recognisable by the patient having difficulty in breathing. This can be recognised by the patient being unable to complete sentences in one breath. A characteristic sign of asthma is that respiration is accompanied by a noise — a wheeze — when the patient breathes out. This is indicative of a lower airway problem. The patient is often coughing and may become distressed and anxious. Laboured breathing may also be evident by the patient using their accessory muscles of respiration to breathe. The respiration rate may rise and be greater than 25 breaths per minute. The patient will also have a tachycardia.

When an acute severe asthma attack is not treated or managed successfully the patient will become tired and eventually exhausted. The clinical features of this **life threatening** asthma will become apparent by a fall in respiration, the rate will drop to less than 8 breaths per minute and a bradycardia will develop (less than 50 beats per minute). Cyanosis will become apparent and the patient will become confused and lose consciousness.

Management

Medical and drug management of asthma consist of assessing and possibly modifying lifestyle and also taking medicines, most commonly delivered by an inhaler. The most effective way of getting the drug quickly to the affected airways is to inhale it. Asthma management can be considered under two broad categories, aimed at **preventing** an attack, and treatments to **relieve** an attack when it occurs.

Prevention

As asthma attack usually occurs in response to exposure to a 'triggering' agent, the most obvious preventive measure is to avoid any contact with these agents. A list of common agents is shown in *Table 10.1*.

Some patients will use 'preventer' inhalers. These are usually red, brown or orange and contain a low dose of steroids and are used regularly — every day. These inhalers work by reducing the swelling and inflammation that occurs when the airways are exposed to a triggering agent, thus reducing the severity of the response. If these inhalers are ineffective at helping to prevent attacks a patient may be prescribed tablets such as a leukotriene receptor antagonist, which mediate the allergic response to the triggering agent.

Table 10.1   Possible triggering agents for asthma

Exposure to allergens (e.g. air pollutants, animal fur, pollen, house dust mites, moulds and fungi, certain foods, medicines such as aspirin and other non-steroidal anti-inflammatory analgesics)
Colds and viral infections
Emotions (particularly stress)
Exercise
Smoking
Hormones
Weather (damp, windy, very cold air)

Bronchodilators

The basic method of relief from an acute asthma attack is to use a drug that has a direct effect on the smooth muscle in the walls of the airways causing it to dilate, thus widening the airway and relieving the constriction. These are called 'bronchodilators', and the most commonly used ones contain salbutamol or terbutaline. Most asthmatics carry their bronchodilator inhalers or 'relievers' with them and they are usually blue. There should always be a blue inhaler in the surgery emergency drug box and this should be readily available for use if necessary. Two puffs should be administered (the dose of salbutamol is 100µg per puff). If the amount of the drug that is absorbed via the inhaler is insufficient to relieve the symptoms then a spacer device can be used in conjunction with an inhaler (shown in *Figure 10.2*). A spacer allows a more effective distribution of the inhaled drug to the lungs and it does not rely on

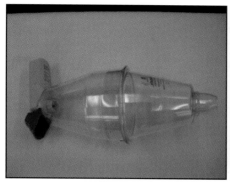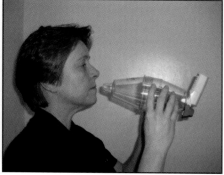

Figure 10.2 Spacer device, and spacer device in use.

coordinating inspiration with the activation of the inhaler. The Resuscitation Council recommends that dental practices should purchase a spacer device. Alternatively, a nebuliser may be used. Commercial nebulisers are available but small disposable chambers can be purchased cheaply and can be attached to an existing oxygen supply for use. These devices effectively create a 'mist' of damp air containing a higher dose of the bronchodilator (usually salbutamol 2.5-5.0mg), which increases the dose getting through to the lungs.

Patients who are having a severe asthma attack which is not responding to standard doses of inhalers should be admitted to hospital for more aggressive treatment. Whilst waiting for the ambulance the patient should be receiving oxygen. If a patient has suffered a prolonged or particularly severe attack they may be prescribed a short course of oral steroids (e.g. prednisolone), which reduces the inflammatory response.

Prevention of an Asthma Attack

It is always sensible to ask a patient who has asthma if it is well controlled and if they know of any triggers that will precipitate an asthma attack. The patient's medication is often a reliable indicator as to how severe a patient's asthma is. Patients who only occasionally use a bronchodilator are likely not to be troubled too much by asthma. Severe asthmatics are on inhalers and tablets and may even have nebulisers at home. One helpful question is to ask if the patient has ever been admitted to hospital with their asthma.

Triggers should be avoided, and those of particular significance in a dental surgery or connected with dental treatment include flowers and plants in the waiting room, pain, stress if a patient is worried about treatment, and analgesics (prescribed or over the counter preparations) that may have been taken for pain relief, in particular aspirin and other non-steroidal anti-inflammatory drugs such as ibuprofen. If stress is a known trigger and the patient is anxious about dental treatment then the dentist should consider appropriate pain and anxiety control measures. This may involve the use of sedation for certain dental procedures.

It is unwise to undertake elective dental treatment if a patient's airway is compromised, for example they have a chest infection. If a patient is breathless from rushing to the surgery they should be allowed to relax until their breathing rate is normal before treatment is undertaken. If a patient is of the opinion that they would benefit from using their inhaler at the start of treatment then this should be allowed. It is not unusual for a dentist to ask a patient, who uses their inhaler regularly, if they would like to use their reliever inhaler at the start of every treatment session. The inhaler should also be readily available.

CHAPTER 11

Cardiovascular Accidents and Transient Ischaemic Attacks

DEFINITION
A cerebrovascular accident — or stroke — is a sudden attack of weakness affecting one side of the body due to an interruption of blood flow to a part of the brain; the signs and symptoms do not resolve within 24 hours

PREDISPOSING FACTORS
- Hypertension
- Diabetes
- Obesity
- Heart disease
- Renal disease
- Previous TIA/CVA
- Atrial fibrillation
- Increased clotting tendencies
- Poor diet
- Smoking
- Excess alcohol consumption
- Age (most people affected are over 65 years old)

SIGNS AND SYMPTOMS (*these can vary considerably*)
- Paralysis of one side of the face
- Paralysis of the limbs on one side
- Confusion
- Inability to speak
- Visual disturbances
- Unilateral tingling
- Unilateral numbness
- Seizures
- Sudden onset of severe headache
- Sudden onset of coma

MANAGEMENT
- Assess ABCDE
- Give oxygen
- Call emergency services
- Reassure the patient is conscious
- Monitor ABCDE

A cerebrovascular accident (CVA), colloquially known as a stroke, is the third largest cause of death, and the single biggest cause of severe adult disability in the UK. Approximately 150,000 people have a stroke in the UK each year. Cardiovascular accidents account for around 1 in 15 deaths in the developed world with the majority being caused by atherosclerosis of a cerebral blood vessel. A CVA is a brain injury and occurs when a part of the brain is damaged or dies because it has been deprived of its essential blood supply.

A transient ischaemic attack (TIA) is also called a mini-stroke and is caused by a temporary loss of blood supply to part of the brain. A TIA presents with symptoms similar to those of a stroke but these usually do not last very long and resolve within 24 hours with the patient making a complete recovery. However around 20% of people who experience a TIA will suffer a full CVA within four weeks, therefore TIAs should be regarded as a warning sign that further TIAs or a complete stroke may occur.

KEY POINT

A transient ischaemic attack is the result of a temporary disruption of blood flow to a part of the brain. Symptoms maybe similar to a stroke but patients recover within 24 hours.

Physiology

The blood supply to the brain is well developed and plentiful and is supplied by the internal carotid and vertebral arteries. Approximately one fifth of the circulating blood volume supplies the brain. All CVAs result from a loss of blood supply to an area of the brain and results in the death of brain cells (neurones). The result is a focal neurological deficit of vascular origin. There are two types of cerebrovascular accident:

Thromboembolic CVA
This is caused by a blood vessel supplying part of the brain becoming blocked by the presence of a atheromatous plaque or less commonly a blood clot (an embolus). The part of the brain that is supplied by that vessel does not receive any blood supply and therefore dies — resulting in an infarction. Thromboembolic CVAs account for approximately 85% of all strokes. The sequence of events causing the narrowing of blood vessel from atherosclerosis is similar to the cause described for a myocardial infarction.

KEY POINT

The UK Stroke Association promotes the use of a short and easily remembered acronym to help the public act fast to assess whether someone has had a stroke. This is FAST:

F — Facial weakness: can the person smile?
A — Arm weakness: can the person raise both arms?
S — Speech problems: can the person speak clearly?
T — Test all three: If the person has any difficulty dial 999

Haemorrhagic CVA

This is less frequent than ischaemic CVAs and is caused by a cerebral blood vessel bursting. This leads to a lack of blood supply to a part of the brain and pressure building up within the brain cavity caused by the leaking blood. The pressure also affects other areas of the brain in addition to the original area.

The brain controls everything we do therefore if part of it becomes dysfunctional then activities that we normally take for granted, such as balance, movement, sight, hearing, speech, understanding and memory, can be seriously affected.

A stroke can be fatal. The prognosis for stroke patients is variable, but the mortality rate is around 30% when a stroke is caused by cerebrovascular thrombosis, and to 80% when caused by a cerebral haemorrhage.

There are several predisposing factors that can increase an individual's susceptibility to a CVA and include hypertension, diabetes, and atrial fibrillation. Lifestyle factors such as diet, smoking and alcohol consumption are also important risk factors.

Symptoms and Signs

The clinical features of a stroke can vary considerably and they are dependent upon the area of the brain that has lost its blood supply and also on which side of the brain. The diagnosis of a stroke can therefore be difficult.

The clinical presentation of a CVA is sudden and rapidly progressing and can consist from mild confusion or difficulty in speaking to catastrophic symptoms such as hemiplegia and even cardiac arrest. When a patient presents with any of the symptoms described in the *Key Point* above it is essential that a CVA is considered as a possible cause and the patient is referred to hospital immediately if it is suspected. To ensure best outcome for a patient active treatment in a specialist hospital unit needs to be instigated within 3 hours of the attack occurring.

Management

The dental management of patients who have had a CVA is restricted to assessing and monitoring ABCDE (airways, breathing, circulation, disability, exposure) and the provision of high-flow oxygen, together with an immediate call to the paramedics to facilitate transfer to a specialist unit.

If loss of consciousness has resulted then the patient should be placed in the recovery position if they are breathing. If they are not breathing and have no pulse then cardiopulmonary resuscitation (CPR) should be started immediately. If the patient is conscious then they will need to be reassured as to what is happening and monitored and supported until the paramedics arrive. It is worth remembering that although they may not be able to speak they will probably be able to understand what is happening and they will be extremely frightened. A calm management approach is essential. It is also helpful to ensure that the patient's relatives can be contacted to explain what has happened and to which hospital the patient is being taken to.

Prevention of CVAs and TIAs

The dental team can do little to prevent a CVA or TIA from happening. The medical history can identify predisposing factors in identifying patients who have an increased risk from a CVA. Patients who have had a CVA or TIA within the past 6 months are at a greater risk of having another cerebrovascular event. It is therefore necessary to carry out a risk assessment be decide if elective treatment should be carried out or if the treatment should be deferred by 6 months.

CHAPTER 12

Epilepsy

DEFINITION

Epilepsy describes a group of chronic neurological conditions that present as seizures

PREDISPOSING FACTORS

- Non-compliance with medication
- Stress, anxiety, pain
- Recent changes in medication
- Flickering lights
- Some medication and recreational drugs
- Poorly controlled epilepsy
- Concurrent infection or illness
- Menstruation
- Fasting
- Sleep deprivation

SIGNS AND SYMPTOMS (*presentation can be variable and depends upon the type of epilepsy the patient has. A tonic-clonic seizure is described below*)

- Short periods of absence with full awareness
- Unprovoked smells, fear, extreme emotion
- Short episodes of muscle stiffness or weakness
- Sudden loss of consciousness (may give a cry) usually no movements initially (tonic phase)
- May be bladder incontinence
- May be confused post-seizure

MANAGEMENT

- If tonic-clonic seizure protect patient from harm
- Administer oxygen
- Try to time the duration of the seizure
- Monitor ABC
- Reassure the patient as they are regaining consciousness
- Allow time for recovery and discharge the patient into the care of an escort
- If seizures last longer than 5 minutes, suspect *status epilepticus* and ring for the paramedics. Consider administering 10mg of transmucosal midazolam
- Monitor ABC

PAEDIATRIC DRUG DOSES

- Transmucosal midazolam

  > 10 years: 10mg

  5–10 years: 7.5mg

  1–5 years: 5 mg
- The parents/carers may administer their own rescue medication which may be rectal diazepam or Epistatus® (buccal midazolam gel). In this case they will use a dose they have been prescribed

Epilepsy is a general term for a whole range of conditions that cause a chronic brain disorder, and it is characterised by recurrent, and often unprovoked seizures (fits). Epilepsy affects around 0.4-1% of the population. A seizure is caused by a sudden burst of inappropriate electrical activity originating from a specific area of the brain that causes the brain messages to be temporarily interrupted, halted or mixed up. There are many different types of seizure (approximately 40) and the effects may vary from a brief 'absent' moment (used to be described as *petit-mal* epilepsy), through loss of consciousness to falling to the floor and having tonic-clonic convulsions (used to be described as *grand mal* epilepsy).

Physiology

The clinical presentation of a seizure is dependent upon which area of the brain is affected by the outburst of electrical activity. Seizures are convulsive events that result from abnormal, involuntary neuronal discharges in the cerebral cortex of the brain; this electrical nervous activity may or may not result in a loss of consciousness. Seizures are described as partial when they involve only one area of the brain, and generalised if they involve the whole brain. Partial seizures can develop into generalised seizures if the epileptic activity spreads out across the whole brain area.

Partial seizures are described as either simple (when a patient remains fully conscious and aware of what is happening), or complex (where the patients consciousness is affected and that are unaware of where they are or what they are doing). The effects of a simple partial seizure vary depending on which lobe of the brain is the originating focus. Patients may experience visual disturbances, stiffening of one part of the body, abnormal sensations such as tingling, and one particular form of partial simple seizure that originates in the temporal lobe can cause intense feelings of fear or happiness, often accompanied by strange smells e.g. burning (these sensations are called 'aura' and in patients who progress on to generalized epilepsy will give warning of an imminent attack). Although the effects of partial seizures are of short duration they still can cause considerable distress to patients, and if the seizures are complex the patient will have no memory of what has taken place.

Generalised seizures involve the whole brain and the commonest presentation of these types of seizures is when the patient loses consciousness and falls to the floor and exhibits tonic-clonic contractions, resulting in uncoordinated jerky movements which can be accompanied by voiding of the bladder or bowels. The tonic phase is caused by a synchronous contraction of all the muscles so the patient becomes very stiff, breathing becomes irregular and noises and cries may be audible as the contraction of the respiratory muscles forces air out of the lungs and over the vocal cords. This is followed by the clonic phase where all the muscles independently relax and contract which produces the jerky phase of uncoordinated movements accompanied by profuse salivation, bruxism and occasionally vomiting. Shortly after this phase all movement ceases, the person is deeply unconscious and unresponsive. Recovery is gradual and can take a considerable time — usually between 10 and 15 minutes although it may take longer. This is the postictal phase. It may take an individual up to 2 hours for their cognitive function to return to normal following a seizure. Epileptic seizures are usually short, lasting less than 5 minutes.

When the patient does not enter the recovery phase, following a tonic-clonic seizure, then it is likely that the patient is developing *status epilepticus,* this is a potentially life threatening condition as the patient is at risk of exhaustion, hypoglycaemia, brain damage due to cerebral hypoxia and cardiac arrest. The patient needs to be transferred to hospital as soon as possible. The incidence of *status epilepticus* amongst epileptic patients is around 5% and the condition carries an acute mortality rate of 10%. The most common precipitating factor for *status epilepticus* is patients failing to comply with their medication regimen.

KEY POINT

Status epilepticus **is defined as a general convulsion lasting 30 minutes or longer, or can be repeated tonic-clonic convulsions occurring over a 30 minute period without recovery of consciousness between each convulsion. In clinical practice any convulsive phase of a tonic-clonic seizure that lasts in excess of 5 minutes should be treated as** *status epilepticus.*

Signs and Symptoms

Considering the numerous types of epilepsy it is hardly surprising that a seizure may present with a variety of signs and symptoms. The patient, their close family and friends or carers should be familiar with these. A generalised tonic-clonic seizure should be quite straight forward to recognise, especially given a patient's medical history. Some patients may have an 'aura' phase and be able to warn you that they are about to have a seizure. The dental team may witness the following over a period of a few minutes:

- A sudden loss of consciousness and if they are standing they will fall to the floor. The patient may cry out. The patient may become cyanotic at this stage. This is the tonic phase of the seizure
- Within less than a minute the patient should have jerking movement of the limbs due to muscle contractions. This is the clonic phase and they might bite their tongue
- Bladder emptying may occur and frothing of the mouth may be seen
- After a period of a few minutes (usually less than 5 minutes) the patient will become relaxed but may remain unconscious. During their recovery they may be confused (post-ictal confusion) and uncertain as to where they are and what has happened.

If the patient is having repeated seizures or one seizure is lasting longer than 5 minutes then it is likely that the patient will go in to *status epilepticus.*

Precipitating Factors

There can be many factors that can precipitate seizures and some examples are given in *Table 12.1*

Table 12.1   Factors which may precipitate epileptic seizures

Withdrawal or failure to take anticonvulsant medication
medication which is eliptogenic (for example, tricyclics, some anaesthetic agents, alcohol)
Sleep deprivation and fatigue
Infection
Pyrexia
Stress
Starvation and hypoglycaemia
Menstruation
Flickering lights
Monotonous tones/sounds

Management

All treatment must be stopped immediately irrespective of the nature of the seizure. It is very important to note the time the seizure started and to monitor its duration. The main focus of management is to protect the patient from harm, remove all sharp objects and ensure that the patient cannot bang themselves on any adjacent equipment. Pillows or blankets may be used to cover immovable objects on which the person may injure themselves, such as the spittoon. Do not attempt to restrain the patient or to put anything in their mouth (such as an airway or mouth prop) whilst they are fitting. If a patient reports an aura, which may precede a tonic-clonic seizure, it is a good idea to position them on the floor, surrounded by cushions or pillows to ensure they are protected prior to the full seizure starting. If possible administer high flow oxygen, and if they are not having tonic-clonic seizures (or when these have finished) maintain the patient in the recovery position to encourage drainage of saliva and vomit away from the airways. Continue to monitor ABC (airways, breathing, circulation), but ensure the patients movements are not inhibited as this can result in them being injured.

All staff must be aware of their own safety also and ensure they are not in a position where they could be inadvertently bitten or kicked.

Once the seizure has finished continue to monitor ABC and maintain oxygen support until the patient has recovered. Allow the patient to recover quietly and slowly and ensure the environment is controlled and private to ensure the patient's dignity is maintained. It is important that all staff appreciate the importance of gentle reassurance and understanding of the patient's disorientation and confusion in the immediate recovery phase.

When the patient has recovered sufficiently they can go home with a suitable escort; they should not be discharged unaccompanied, and a competent adult should stay with them for some hours afterwards. It is not usually necessary to send a patient to hospital following a seizure. The patient should only be transferred to hospital if their seizure was atypical, they developed *status epilepticus*, or the patients injured themselves during the seizure.

When a seizure continues for longer than 5 minutes, or there are repetitive seizures for greater than 5 minutes, there is a danger of *status epilepticus* developing. When *status epilepticus* is suspected the emergency services must be called and the patient transferred to hospital. Other than high flow oxygen the only other interventive treatment to be considered for *status epilepticus* is the administration of 10mg of midazolam by a transmucosal route — buccal or intranasal. Paramedics may administer rectal diazepam, intra-venous diazepam or midazolam.

When managing children with *status epilepticus* the parent or carer may use their own rescue medication which may be rectal diazepam or buccal midazolam gel. These carers will have been informed of what dose to give. The dose of benzodiazepines given to children is usually calculated by weight, but this is often not feasible in a dental surgery. The doses of transmucosal midazolam advised by the Resuscitation Council (UK) for children who have *status epilepticus* are 10mg if they are over 10 years of age; 7.5mg for 5-10 year old's, and 5mg for children between 1-5 years old.

Prevention of Seizures

As for all dental patients a full medical history is essential but it is always essential to have a record of detailed information from any patient with a history of seizures. If the patient themselves cannot provide this history it should be elicited from their carers. The nature of the condition can change, with patients having 'good' or 'bad' phases with respect to their epilepsy. This history should therefore be updated before each visit as the pattern of the illness might have changed. The following information should be obtained from patients who suffer from epilepsy in order that a risk assessment can be undertaken:

- The type of seizures experienced by the patient and their duration
- How well controlled are the seizures and how often do they occur and when was the last seizure
- How does the patient normally recover from a seizure and how long does this process usually take
- Are there any triggers that may precipitate a seizure and does the patient usually have any warning that they are going to have a seizure
- Has the patient ever had *status epilepticus*, and if so how many times
- Has the patient taken their anti-epileptic medication as usual and has the type of medication prescribed changed recently

The answers to the above questions will help the dental team assess the likelihood of a seizure occurring in the dental surgery and how best to recognise and manage it. If a patient with dental anxiety knows that stress is a trigger for their seizures then the team must consider if it is more appropriate to treat the patient under sedation. If a patient has recently changed their anti-epileptic medication or their seizure control is poor the patient is likely to be at an increased risk of having a seizure.

Low blood sugar levels can precipitate an attack so taking a blood glucose reading before treatment may be advisable for some patients; if the reading is less than 3mmol/l then glucose should be given before treatment.

CHAPTER 13

Faints

DEFINITION

Loss of consciousness caused by a temporary insufficient blood supply to the brain

PREDISPOSING FACTORS

- Prolonged standing
- Prolonged exposure to heat
- Stress/anxiety
- Sudden extreme emotion
- Nausea and vomiting
- Fasting
- Dehydration
- Painful stimuli or unpleasant stimuli (e.g. watching someone experience pain)

SIGNS AND SYMPTOMS

- Feeling hot and sweaty
- Pallor
- Auditory and visual disturbances
- Light headed or dizzy
- Slow pulse (bradycardia)
- Brief loss of consciousness
- Tonic-clonic movements can occur

MANAGEMENT

- Avoid triggers if possible
- Immediately place in supine position but have head down and elevate legs
- Administer high flow oxygen (6–8l/min)
- Monitor ABC
- Reassure patient
- Upon recovery return the patient to the upright position gradually

PAEDIATRIC DRUG DOSES

Doses of any medication are the same as above

A faint is also called syncope, vasovagal syncope or vasovagal attack. The word syncope means a sudden loss of consciousness, and vasovagal is referring to the action of the vagus nerve in causing a faint (see explanation below). Faints are a common occurrence; 50% of the population will experience a faint at least once during their lifetime, and 3% of the population suffer from recurrent episodes. Whilst fainting is rarely life-threatening it is extremely unpleasant for the patient and can continue to cause them to feel unwell for several hours afterwards. It is also important to remember that the sudden loss of consciousness can also result in patients injuring themselves if they fall to the floor.

There can be some pathological causes of syncope, for example some cardiac causes, which would need to be excluded if a patient is having repeated episodes.

A faint is usually initiated by a predisposing factor or trigger and some of these are given in *Table 13. 1*. The stimuli that may precipitate a faint can be physical or psychological. The most common triggers in a dental surgery setting are stress or anxiety and pain. Most people will realise that they are not feeling normal before a faint and there are symptoms leading up to the loss of consciousness. Faints can sometimes be aborted if action is taken early enough.

Physiology

The trigger produces a direct or indirect effect on a particular area of the brain stem in the central nervous system (CNS) and this leads to an increased activity of the parasympathetic nervous system, which includes the vagus nerve. This increased vagal activity causes a drop in heart rate and a significant drop in blood pressure. There is also a reduction

Table 13.1   Triggers for vasovagal syncope

Prolonged standing or sitting upright	Sudden extreme emotion
Stress/anxiety	Hunger or fasting
Painful stimuli	Nausea and vomiting
Unpleasant stimuli (for example watching someone experiencing pain)	Dehydration
Prolonged exposure to heat	

in sympathetic nervous system activity causing a dilatation of the blood vessels leading to increased 'pooling' of the blood volume in the limbs. This pooling of blood peripherally reduces the volume of blood entering the heart and leads to a further drop in blood pressure. All this means there is less blood flowing to the brain and it results in cerebral hypoxia and unconsciousness. As one of the main contributing factors to the faint is the pooling of blood in the lower limbs the effects can be reversed very rapidly by lying the patient flat and elevating the legs, thus encouraging the blood to return to the heart which will increase the stroke volume (and hence the cardiac output), increase the blood pressure and thus reduce the cerebral hypoxia.

Symptoms and Signs

The fundamental effect on the body is that of cerebral hypoxia, which is progressive, so there are frequently several prodromal symptoms and signs that provide warning of impending loss of consciousness. A person who has fainted previously will recognise these and be alerted to the fact that they are about to faint again. A person who is experiencing a primary event may not be aware of what is happening but may well vocalise some of the symptoms and will show obvious signs of the impending episode.

The symptoms vary between individuals but include initially feeling very warm and light headed, the patient will be very pale and sweaty, they may notice distortion of sounds (voices sound very far away) and loss of visual acuity, and their pulse rate will be very slow which is a useful diagnostic tool. After a few seconds they will lose consciousness and will collapse towards the floor if they are standing, or lean over if they are sitting up.

As soon as the blood flow to the brain is restored they will recover consciousness with full awareness of their surroundings, although they will continue to feel unwell for some time afterwards. It should be remembered that if a patient is propped upright, for example in a chair, then cerebral blood flow will not be returned and this can lead to death if the circulation is not restored.

Management

When a patient becomes very pale and loses consciousness they should immediately be placed flat with leg elevated (above the level of the heart) and oxygen administered. This will help to restore the cerebral oxygen concentration more quickly. As the patient begins to recover leave them in this position for several minutes before returning them, very slowly, to an upright-seated posture. Reassure the patient as they are likely to feel embarrassed and may be uncertain as to what happened. It is helpful to monitor the pulse rate because there will be an increase in the rate as recovery starts, and after a minute the rate may become quite rapid but will stabilise to normal very quickly. A pulse oximeter can be a useful aid if one is available.

In profound faints it is possible to get spontaneous muscle movements that may mimic a seizure, and occasionally bladder emptying may occur. The pulse rate will provide the diagnosis here if there is concern as to the diagnosis — with a seizure the pulse rate will be very rapid, with a faint it will be very slow.

A patient who is pregnant and has fainted still needs to be placed supine but they must be positioned on their side, otherwise the weight of the uterus pressing onto the inferior vena cava will prevent the blood returning to the heart effectively and the circulation will not be restored. It is usual to lay the patient on their left side — pillows or a person may be required to maintain the patient in this position whilst they are unconscious.

Prevention

The best form of management is avoidance, and therefore it is always useful to know what the triggers are if someone has a history of fainting. Ensuring that the patient is adequately hydrated and has a good blood sugar level (i.e. has eaten recently) can help to minimise the likelihood of a faint. It is very rare for patients to faint when lying down because it is impossible for blood to pool in the limbs. It may be helpful to carry out the dental examination and administration of local anaesthetic with a patient supine if they are nervous or stressed about these aspects of treatment. As soon as a patient complains of feeling hot or dizzy then immediate action is needed to prevent progression by stopping treatment immediately, altering the chair position to flat. Putting a fan on (or opening a window) will help to avert a full blown faint. Do remember to reassure the patient and explain what you are doing otherwise they may become more stressed.

When stress and anxiety associated with dental treatment causes a faint then the value of using sedation for treatments that the patient perceives as stressful should be considered.

CHAPTER 14

Hyperventilation and Panic Attacks

DEFINITION
Breathing at an abnormally rapid rate whilst at rest

PREDISPOSING FACTORS
- Stress and anxiety
- Pain
- Chronic generalised anxiety disorder

SIGNS AND SYMPTOMS
- Rapid shallow breathing
- Gasping and Struggling to breathe
- Tingling of mouth and fingers and limbs
- Dizziness
- Muscle spasms, pain and rigidity (tetanic cramps)
- Chest pain
- Tachycardia and palpitations
- Extreme distress
- Loss of consciousness

MANAGEMENT
- Reassurance
- Place in a comfortable position and ensure the patient has some privacy, if possible
- Try to reduce anxiety
- Encourage patient to try and slow down the breathing rate
- Encourage re-breathing through cupped hands or paper bag to reverse alkalosis
- Allow recovery

Hyperventilation is literally 'overbreathing' — when a patient is taking rapid panting breaths in a situation where this type of breathing is not required. Obviously if a person is undertaking extreme exercise they will breathe rapidly, but in these circumstances the body is demanding extra oxygen and the respiratory system is responding to this demand and this is not hyperventilation.

Physiology

Blood is a slightly alkaline fluid with a pH of 7.4, and this needs to be maintained for optimum functioning of all the body's metabolic processes. A decreased or low pH is called an 'acidosis' and a rise in pH is called an 'alkalosis'. When the blood pH exceeds 7.8 or falls below 7.0 all processes cease and the body will die. It is therefore not surprising that there are several regulatory mechanisms in place to try and maintain an optimum blood, tissue and cell pH. This is also referred to as the acid-base balance.

Respiration is an important system in the maintenance of blood pH because the level of carbon dioxide in the body has a direct effect on blood pH. The carbon dioxide combines with water to form carbonic acid which then splits into two separate components, a hydrogen ion and a bicarbonate ion:

$$H_2O + CO_2^- = H_2CO_3^- = H^+ + HCO_3^-$$

The hydrogen ion concentration is very important and if there is a reduction in carbon dioxide there will be less hydrogen ions produced, which will cause the blood pH to rise producing an alkalosis. This begins to have an effect on the body's metabolism and one of the earliest things adversely affected is the drop in the available level of calcium to be used by the nervous system. Calcium is required to regulate the excitability of the nerves. If a person hyperventilates they 'blow off' far too much carbon dioxide, this raises the blood pH and lowers the calcium concentration, resulting in muscle spasms and sensory disturbances such as tingling.

Symptoms and Signs

Hyperventilation produces a variety of symptoms including dizziness, weakness, tinnitus, sweating, tingling sensations around the lips and extremities of the limbs, muscle spasms and cramps, tachycardia, palpitations, and chest pain. Loss of consciousness is very uncommon, but can occur.

Carpopedal spasm — spasm of the hands and feet — may be observed. This is caused by the reduction in the blood calcium level.

Management

It is essential to reduce the rate and increase the depth of respiration. Reassure the patient and gently and quietly exert a calming influence by asking them to concentrate on breathing slowly. The patient's carbon dioxide levels can further be raised by asking them to hold their breath for as long as possible, or by 're-breathing' their expired air as this has a higher carbon dioxide level than room air. The simplest re-breathing method is to ask the patient to breathe in and out of their cupped hands that are placed around their nose and mouth. Alternatively the patient can breathe into a paper bag whilst being encouraged to breathe slowly, although some authorities suggest that there is a risk of hypoxia with this method. As the carbon dioxide level rises the symptoms will disappear very quickly, especially the sensory symptoms.

It is important to remember that the symptoms are very frightening and distressing for the patient, and they are also often very embarrassed. Not surprisingly this will increase their panic levels and make the situation worse. It is therefore essential to constantly reassure the patient that the symptoms will resolve soon and that nothing serious is happening. If the chest pain remains the patient needs to be assessed by a specialist to exclude underlying cardiac pathology.

Prevention

When the patient is calm it is helpful to explain why hyperventilation happens and to identify the triggers. Sedation may be required to undertake dental treatment for some patients, and referral for behavioural therapy may also be helpful.

Panic Attacks

Situations of extreme fear or stress can result in hyperventilaltion, and this is also one of the symptoms of a panic attack. As a consequence of this it can be very difficult to differentiate whether the patient is suffering a panic attack, or an extreme fear response. To a certain extent this is a semantic argument as the management remains the same, but it is necessary for a healthcare professional to have an understanding of the causes and effects of panic attacks as many patients who attend for dental treatment do suffer from them.

A panic attack is a sudden episode of very intense fear that can occur at any time — it can occur when people are alone, in public, or even when they are asleep. There is often no known trigger. There is no known cause but certain biochemical mediators, heredity and sustained stress are possible predisposing factors.

Panic attacks usually begin very suddenly, reach a maximum intensity after about 10 minutes and then the reaction subsides over the next 30 minutes. However in some patients they can last hours or even days. The symptoms vary but the common ones are listed in *Table 14.1*.

Table 14.1   Symptoms experienced in panic attacks

Rapid heart rate	Tremors
Abdominal cramping	Hyperventilation
Sweating	Chills
Chest pain	Headache
Dizziness	Hot flushes
Faintness	Sense of impending death
Trouble swallowing and 'throat tightness'	Irrational behaviour
Nausea	

Physiology

The normal response to a perceived threat to the body's survival is the 'fight or flight' response which is mediated predominantly by a surge of adrenaline, and is associated with activity within the sympathetic nervous system. The direct actions of an adrenaline surge is to:

- Dilate the pupils, erect body hairs
- Inhibit digestion
- Constrict the arterioles thus producing a rise in blood pressure and dilate the coronary vessels increasing the blood flow to cardiac muscle
- Dilate the bronchioles thus increasing the amount of air movement on inspiration and expiration, and increase the rate and volume of respiration.

The responses listed above are all very useful when they are needed to facilitate rapid movement away from a potential threat, but are not helpful at a person at rest.

Management

The main management method is to use the mind's cognitive powers to reverse the effects by recognising that no specific threat exists. This can be aided by breathing awareness and a deliberate attempt to slow the breathing rate down by taking slow deep breaths and lying down in a semi-reclined position with the eyes closed. Talking quietly and calmly to the patient may be helpful, but some people find this an irritating distraction and it is best to ask the people themselves what they find the most helpful. The attack will gradually subside but the patient will need adequate time to recover completely as these attacks are distressing and can be very tiring. In some patients who suffer prolonged and severe attacks medication may be used to control them.

CHAPTER 15

Hypoglycaemia

DEFINITION

Hypoglycaemia can be defined as an abnormally low level of glucose in the bloodstream

PREDISPOSING FACTORS

- Diabetes
- Fasting
- Anxiety
- The presence of any debilitating disease such as infection

SIGNS AND SYMPTOMS

- Cold and clammy
- Sweating
- Pallor
- Tremor and shaking
- Double vision
- Drowsiness
- Pins and needles in lips and tongue
- Slurred speech
- Behavioural/mood changes (for example, excitable, irritable, aggressive, uncooperative, confusion)
- Loss of consciousness
- Convulsions

MANAGEMENT

Conscious hypoglycaemia

- Give approximately 10–20g glucose by oral route (for example, glucose drink, 200mls milk)
- Use a glucose monitor if available
- Monitor ABC and consider oxygen

Unconscious hypoglycaemia

- 1mg glucagon by intramuscular of subcutaneous injection. Follow with oral glucose when consciousness is recovered
- Monitor and review ABC and consider oxygen
- Call paramedics if necessary
- Use a glucose monitor if one is available

PAEDIATRIC DOSES

> 8 years: use adult doses of glucagon and glucose

< 8 years: 500µg glucagon intramuscular (= 0.5mg)

Hypoglycaemia is a low blood sugar level and the patient may ultimately lose consciousness. However, there are usually several signs and symptoms as the condition is developing and the patient is deteriorating.

Physiology

Glucose is an essential energy source and is required by all of the body's cells — without it cell death ensues. Some of the body's tissues have the ability to store glucose in the form of glycogen (a larger molecule), however, the cells of the nervous system cannot store glucose. Nervous tissue is therefore totally reliant on the glucose available in the bloodstream to maintain normal function. The level of glucose in the blood needs to be between 60-100mg of glucose per 100ml of blood for optimal cellular function. Blood glucose levels are usually expressed as millimoles per litre, with normal levels being around 3.3–5.5 mmols/l. Chronic abnormal levels of glucose have a long lasting deleterious effects on the body.

Blood glucose levels are derived from carbohydrates ingested as food (see *Figure 15.1*). The carbohydrates are broken down in the digestive tract, and are

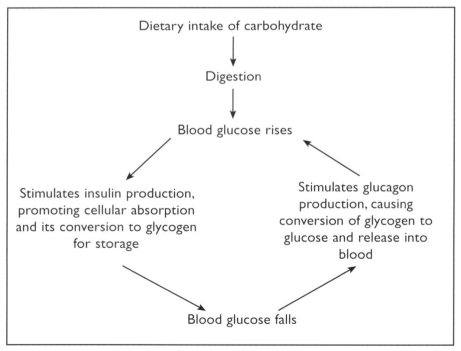

Figure 15.1 The maintenance of blood glucose.

then absorbed into the blood stream. Blood glucose levels are usually tightly controlled, or regulated, so that optimum levels of glucose are maintained in the blood throughout the day, even during the 'fasting' periods. The main regulatory mechanism is through the endocrine system, which produces hormones that are released into the bloodstream to control our metabolism. The pancreas produces two important hormones, **insulin** and **glucagon,** which are essential in the regulation of blood glucose. Insulin facilitates the entry of glucose from the blood into cells, such as the liver, where glucose can be stored as glycogen — an energy source. Glucagon effectively reverses this process by converting the stored liver glycogen back into glucose. This glucose is released into the bloodstream for immediate use.

Hypoglycaemia can result from:

- Insufficient dietary intake of carbohydrate
- Anxiety due to the nervous tissue requiring more energy than normal
- Infection due to the increased metabolic rate utilising more glucose
- Excess insulin being present for the level of glucose in the blood at any particular time.

Symptoms and Signs

A blood glucose of less than 3 mmol/l is usually considered as being indicative of hypoglycaemia. There are some patients who will develop symptoms at a higher level than this. Some adults will know if their blood sugar level is falling and will take carbohydrates to address this. The consequences of a low blood sugar can have a profound and immediate effect on the nervous system and this accounts for many of the symptoms, especially the profound behavioural changes such as irritability, aggression and confusion. Physical changes are also apparent and will include pallor, sweating, tremor and shaking, double vision, drowsiness and ultimately loss of consciousness. A patient who is hypoglycaemic may also exhibit uncontrollable tonic-clonic movements (convulsions/fitting).

Diabetes

A patient with diabetes has lost the ability to naturally regulate their blood glucose levels. In Type I diabetics the pancreas cannot produce insulin at all and therefore when insulin is required it must be injected. Type II diabetics do produce insulin but the insulin is not very effective — there is a cellular resistance to the effects of insulin. Clinically this means that Type II diabetics have, in effect, an insulin deficiency that will be variable depending on the individual patient. Each patient needs to adjust and monitor their diet other wise they may need to take medication to help control their glucose levels. It is therefore essential that all diabetic patients monitor their blood glucose levels carefully and take appropriate action to maintain normal glucose levels. This is achieved by regularly measuring blood glucose using a finger prick test (a small drop of blood is absorbed onto a test stick). This is then inserted into a machine that measures the glucose concentration.

Management

The treatment for hypoglycaemia is to increase the circulating blood glucose levels, and there are three ways of doing this:

1. Oral intake of carbohydrate
This is only possible in a conscious patient and the dental team needs to ensure that around 10–20g of glucose is given in any convenient form available. The following are suitable:-

- Glucose gel*
- Three sugar cubes or two teaspoons of sugar
- Chocolate bars
- 200ml milk
- 50–55ml sparkling glucose drink

* The proprietary glucose gel available is administered into the buccal sulcus and is quickly absorbed transmucosally (across the vascular oral mucosa).

2. Injection of glucagon
This hormone will increase the blood glucose levels by stimulating the conversion of glycogen into glucose. It is usually used in the unconscious hypoglycaemic patient and administered by intramuscular (IM) or subcutaneous (SC) injection, although it can also be given intravenously (however this is unlikely to be the case in the majority of dental surgeries). The dose is 1mg and the proprietary preparations available all contain this dose. Glucagon is very short-acting so when the patient recovers consciousness they should be given oral carbohydrates as soon as possible in order to sustain blood glucose levels.

3. Infusion of a glucose solution directly into the bloodstream

This is not usually practical to do in a dental surgery environment as dental staff are unlikely to have the necessary expertise to gain intravenous access and administer a slow infusion of 25ml of a 50% solution of dextrose. However paramedics may do this.

Prevention

It is important to ensure that suitable appointment times are made for known diabetics so as to avoid disruption of the patients' normal meal times. It should be acknowledged that anxiety and infection both increase glucose demand and may precipitate unexpected hypoglycaemia. Patients who are diabetic should be asked if they have taken their medication and food as usual and when their next food and diabetic medication is due. When patients have chronic poorly controlled diabetes, enquiries should be made as how regularly the patient experiences low blood sugar levels or 'hypos', and the dental team need to be aware and alert to this possibility occurring. Additional information and often reassurance can be quickly obtained by measuring a patient's blood glucose. Devices to measure blood glucose are relatively inexpensive and are quick and easy to use. The Resuscitation Council (UK) advised in 2006 that dental practices should have an automated blood glucose measurement device as part of their medical emergency and resuscitation equipment.

Hyperglycaemia

This is defined as abnormally high blood glucose levels and usually occurs in patients with undiagnosed diabetes or poorly controlled Type I diabetes. This condition is much less common than hypoglycaemia. The symptoms of hyperglycaemia are slow to develop and include a chronic thirst, frequent urination, lethargy and increased susceptibility to infection. These symptoms are the same as for undiagnosed or untreated diabetes. If the serum glucose levels become very high then this can appear to induce similar physical signs and symptoms to hypoglycaemia and can eventually lead to coma.

The treatment is hospital admission and carefully monitored administration of insulin. When a diabetic patient becomes unconscious in the dental surgery it is usual to treat the patient for hypoglycaemia, as this is the most likely cause of collapse. It is only when a patient fails to recover and a blood glucose measurement obtained that hyperglycaemia would be suspected. In any event the patient would be transferred to hospital.

In a conscious diabetic patient who felt unwell their history would help to arrive at a diagnosis, and it is likely that the patient has felt unwell for several days. A possible scenario for hyperglycaemia in a diabetic would be that the patient has missed multiple doses of insulin but has eaten as normal.

CHAPTER 16

Rare Causes of Collapse

The emergencies described in the previous chapters are well documented as having occurred in a dental surgery setting, albeit rarely. However there are several other potential causes of collapse that are very rare but are covered in this chapter for completeness.

Adrenal Shock

DEFINITION
Deterioration or collapse of a patient with adrenal insufficiency

PREDISPOSING FACTORS
- Stress in a patient who has adrenal insufficiency because of:
- Primary addison's disease
- Suppression of the adrenal glands from steroid therapy

SIGNS AND SYMPTOMS
- Pallor
- Hypotension
- Loss of consciousness

MANAGEMENT
- Lay the patient flat
- Administer oxygen
- Give 100-200mg hydrocortison intravenous if available
- Call for pramedics; intravenous fluid replacement may be required

This is also called a steroid crisis or an Addisonian crisis. Adrenal shock occurs because the adrenal cortex fails to produce the necessary corticosteroid hormones that enable the body to cope adequately with a stressful situation. This can be due to two main causes:

- Primary failure of the adrenal cortex itself resulting in adrenal insufficiency — this condition is called Addison's disease. Patients suffering from this condition are usually well aware of it and take regular replacement drug therapy to compensate for the deficit in hormones.
- Secondary reduction in adrenal cortex activity. The reduced corticosteroid production is usually a result of a side effect of medication (usually steroids).

Physiology

The glucocorticoid hormones (e.g cortisol) have a wide range of actions including the regulation of the metabolism of carbohydrates, fats and proteins, decreasing the absorption of calcium from the gut, reducing inflammation, reducing the allergic responses of the body and causing some sodium (and hence also water) retention. The secretion of these hormones is diurnal, as they are produced twice per day, and the stimulus for their secretion is falling blood levels. The blood levels are 'monitored' by the pituitary gland and when the levels fall below a certain value the pituitary gland produces a hormone, adrenocorticotrophic hormone (ACTH), which stimulates the adrenal cortex to produce more cortisol. When the body is stressed the higher brain centres stimulate the hypothalamus, which in turn stimulates the pituitary causing the production of ACTH and even more cortisol is produced. As the control of this production responds directly to the circulating level of cortisol, a person who takes synthetic steroids for another condition (e.g. prednisolone to reduce inflammation in arthritis) will have a high level, so the body will produce less of its own steroids. This can mean that the body begins to lose the ability to produce natural cortisol and therefore cannot 'respond' when extra hormone is required (*Figure 16.1*).

Signs and Symptoms

The patient will become very pale, with a rapid weak and thready pulse. The blood pressure drops dramatically and this may result in loss of consciousness and coma.

Management

The management in a dental surgery setting is limited to the provision of high flow oxygen, monitoring ABCDE (airways, breathing, circulation, disability, exposure), and laying the patient flat and elevating the legs to help compensate for the hypotension. The administration of 100mg hydrocortisone sodium succcinate preferably IV, but IM is a possibility, if this drug is available it can be administered. The patient needs to be transferred to hospital as soon as possible.

Prevention

Some authorities recommend that patients who are 'theoretically' at risk of an adrenal crisis, e.g. patients who are on long-term steroid therapy, should

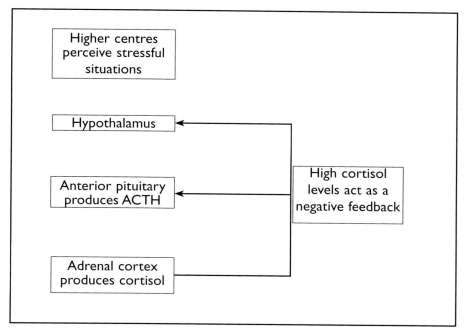

Figure 16.1 Summary of the regulation of blood cortisol levels

increase the circulating levels of glucocorticoids before a potentially stressful situation occurs. This is thought to be important if patients are having major surgery under general anaesthesia. The relevance of adrenal suppression to routine dental practice has been contentious in the past. Extra or prophylactic steroid cover has been administered before dental surgery by increasing the patient's regular oral steroid dose taken on the morning of the procedure. Alternatively, an intramuscular dose can be given just before treatment. There is, however, no evidence base for this practice, and currently it is not a requirement for dental surgeries to carry hydrocortisone in their emergency drug kits, so if a patient has been advised to do this by their medical practitioner this would be done under their supervision and not the dentist.

Drug Overdose

There is evidence to suggest that the use of 'recreational' drugs is increasing and it is possible that a patient attending for dental treatment may be still under the influence of these drugs. The signs and symptoms would be bizarre and inappropriate behaviour, irrational mood swings and alteration in pupil responses may occur. No treatment should be undertaken and the patient should be transferred to a hospital as soon as possible. If a patient is under the influence of alcohol treatment should not be carried out and the patient should be sent home with an escort who will remain with them until the effects have worn off. It is essential to exclude other causes for this behaviour, for example hypoglycaemia, before concluding that drugs or alcohol may be the cause.

There are two drugs that are administered in dental surgeries that can result in collapse due to overdose, these are local anaesthetics and benzodiazepines.

Local Anaesthetics

DEFINITION
The administration of too much drug which has resulted in significant harmful effects
PREDISPOSING FACTORS
• Very young and the elderly
• Pre-existing systemic disease (in particular liver disease and kidney disease)
• Concurrent medication
SIGNS AND SYMPTOMS
• Lightheadedness, visual or hearing disturbances
• Agitation
• Confusion
• Seizures
• Respiratory distress
• Loss of consciousness
• Respiratory and cardiac arrest
MANAGEMENT
• Administer oxygen
• Maintain airway
• Call paramedics
• Monitor ABCDE

Although local anaesthetic agents are very safe it is necessary to remember that if used without due care and attention overdose can occur. The susceptibility of a patient to the toxic side effects will be reduced in the very young, the elderly and patients who have liver or kidney disease, therefore the recommended 'maximum' dose that the manufacturers state in their information leaflets will need to be reduced. The maximum recommended dose for lignocaine is 4.4mg/kg with an absolute ceiling of 300mg. These doses are advisable even if there is a vasoconstrictor present. The 2.2ml cartridge of 2% lignocaine contains 44mg of lignocaine (20mg/ml). *Table 16.1* gives the recommended maximum doses of lignocaine.

Physiology

Local anaesthetic agents are membrane stabilisers and have profound effects on the nervous system. Initially, local anaesthetic agents can have an excitatory effect, but at high concentrations these agents will cause a reduction in heart rate and significant central nervous system (CNS) depression that can lead to collapse, respiratory depression and death. Many local anaesthetic agents also contain adrenaline; conversely increased levels of adrenaline will cause cardiac arrhythmias. The toxic effects of local anaesthetics are reversible when a small amount of solution has been given as the drug will eventually be metabolised and eliminated.

Signs and Symptoms

Toxic levels of local anaesthetic are more likely to occur in young children and the elderly. An intravascular injection will lead to temporary symptoms. The patient will complain initially of feeling dizzy and light-headed, which may be accompanied by sensory disturbances such as tinnitus, tingling and numbness and abnormal taste. Agitation may occur before this progresses onto confusion and drowsiness, followed by loss of consciousness. If a large overdose has occurred the patient may have tonic-clonic convulsions and coma. The cardiovascular symptoms vary depending on whether adrenaline is also present in the local anaesthetic. If adrenaline is present the patient will develop a rapid heart rate and an elevated blood pressure, if it is not then the initial cardiovascular symptoms will be a slow pulse with a low blood pressure. In both cases the heart conducting system will eventually be affected producing abnormal heart rhythms that can lead to a cardiac arrest.

Management

The best management is obviously prevention, and an awareness of the recommended maximum doses is essential. It is always important to keep

Table 16.1   Maximum recommended dose of 2% lignocaine with 1:80,000 adrenaline

Age/weight	Number of cartridges
5 year old	2
70 kg adult	6.8
NB. All cartridge sizes are 2.2ml	

all the used LA cartridges on the side so that all team members know how much has been administered, and it is advisable to stop administration long before the maximum recommended dose is approached. If the patient does develop any of the signs and symptoms, or it is suspected that the maximum dose has been exceeded, the patient needs to be placed flat, oxygen administered and monitor ABCDE. The patient should be transferred to hospital to allow close supervision and cardiac monitoring in case severe arrhythmias develop.

Oversedation with Benzodiazepines

DEFINITION The administration of too much benzodiazepines, which has resulted in significant respiratory distress
PREDISPOSING FACTORS • Elderly • Pre-existing disease (especially respiratory disease) • Concurrent medication: already taking CNS depressants (prescribed or for recreational use) which may interact with the benzodiazepines
SIGNS AND SYMPTOMS • Uncooperative patient • Failure to respond to commands • Fall in oxygen saturation • Cyanosis of the tissues
MANAGEMENT • Oxygen • Improve airway (head-tilt chin lift or jaw thrust) • Consider giving flumazenil • Monitor ABCDE • Call paramedics if no improvement • Consider assistant ventilation if required • If respiratory arrest then follow BLS algorithm

Benzodiazepines are used for anxious patients by clinicians who undertake conscious sedation techniques. These may be given by oral or transmucosal routes but are more commonly administered intravenously as it allows for the dose to be titrated against patient response (ie. the dose is steadily increased until the appropriate level of sedation is obtained). Midazolam is the IV sedative of choice in dental practice. Benzodiazepines are powerful CNS and respiratory depressants so the effects of an overdose will be to produce unconsciousness and reduce respiration. All patients having sedation will be monitored clinically and with a pulse oximeter by a trained assistant, therefore, an overdose should be able to be identified and managed promptly. If the oxygen saturation begins to drop then dental treatment is halted and oxygen administered immediately. Flumazenil may be administered if necessary. The airway should be maximised by a head-tilt chin lift or a jaw thrust. If a respiratory arrest occurs then the patient must be manually ventilated using a bag valve mask and 100% oxygen at a rate of 12 breaths per minute — airway adjuncts may be helpful. Flumazenil (500μg) should be given, if it has not previously been administered, and the patient supported and monitored until the effects have been completely reversed. Paramedics should be called as the patient should be monitored for several hours. It is essential to remember that the reversal agent does not last in the circulation as long as the benzodiazepine, and therefore as it wears off the patient may become sedated again.

CHAPTER 17

Transfer to the Paramedics

When a patient is in need of emergency specialist treatment the paramedics will transfer them to an accident and emergency department. In order to ensure that this transfer takes place as rapidly and effectively as possible the members of the dental team have a vital role to play in informing the paramedics of the events that took place prior to the emergency and also how the emergency was managed. Failure to give the paramedics essential information may adversely affect the patient's emergency care and waste valuable time. This chapter equips the reader with important information that will optimise the patient's care and outcome.

Step 1 — The Initial Telephone Call

It is important to remember that information given by telephone to the emergency services needs to be stated clearly and calmly. This will avoid misunderstanding and the necessity for repetition. The first action to be taken is to contact the emergency services by dialling 999. This call will be answered by an operator, who will ask you which service you require; you need to specify the ambulance service. The call will then be passed to an ambulance controller who will dispatch the paramedic team. The information you provide to the controller will determine the priority given to the call and thus the speed of the response units.

There are two types of response vehicles: a full paramedic ambulance, which is essentially a mini A&E department with drugs and equipment necessary to deal with most immediate life threatening emergencies, and a rapid response vehicle. The latter may be a car or a motorcycle driven by a single paramedic who carries with them a limited amount of emergency equipment. A rapid response vehicle can arrive in approximately 8 minutes, whereas a paramedic ambulance may take up to 30 minutes, and priority is given to cardio-respiratory arrest. It is therefore essential that the controller receives as much information as possible about the situation.

During the management of a medical emergency someone from the dental team needs to update ambulance control if the situation deteriorates whilst a surgery is waiting for the paramedic to arrive. It is essential to telephone again to 'upgrade' the call. The information required will be the address and location of the surgery; the name and age of the patient, a concise history of the emergency and the likely diagnosis if known, and the current condition of the patient.

Step 2 — Waiting for the Paramedics

It is good practice to note the time the emergency call was made, as this will provide a reference as to how long it is likely to be before professional help arrives. A person should be directed to stand by the front entrance to meet the paramedics and direct them to the location of the patient. This is of paramount importance in premises that have multiple facilities and users. Another member of the team should collect documentation together, ready to give to the paramedics, including all the details and information suggested below.

Step 3 — Transfer of the Patient

The primary role of the paramedics is to transport the patient to a definitive care centre as quickly as possible; however, they will make a rapid assessment of the patient's status and intervene if necessary before transferring the patient. Interventive procedures may need to be undertaken in the dental surgery to stabilise the patient before moving them. Procedures carried out could include any of the following: defibrillation, securing the airway including intubation, setting up an intravenous or intraosseous infusion and administering emergency drugs.

There are several important and possibly vital facts that the paramedics will need to be told upon their arrival, and it is preferable to give them a written account of events also as these can then be added to the patient's A&E records. The important information can be summarised by the acronyms SAMPLE or MAPLES as explained below:

- **S**ymptoms
- **A**llergies
- **M**edications
- **P**ast medical history
- **L**ast oral intake
- **E**vents prior to the incident.

Symptoms
This includes all symptoms and signs that have been noted during the ABCDE assessment of the patient and any interventions carried out by the dental team. The following is essential information:

- Pulse — was it present throughout and what rate (fast or slow?)
- Breathing — was it present throughout and what rate?
- Was the patient conscious or unconscious?
- Was there any pain, where was it located and how severe and how long did it last?
- Did the patient have a seizure?
- What emergency treatment was carried out including were any emergency drugs administered?

Allergies

The potential problem of an allergic reaction is always possible for any practitioner who administers drugs or fluids — the worst-case scenario is that of an anaphylaxis. All the patient's known allergies should be reported to the paramedics. Whilst the allergy may have no direct bearing on the patient's acute condition it may be relevant to the patient's management.

Medications

If at all possible, the patient's medications should be collected together and handed over to the paramedic's upon their arrival. This may not be feasible in a dental surgery setting but a comprehensive drug history should be given to the paramedics at handover. Medications will give vital information to the emergency team regarding pre-existing medical conditions that the patient may not be fully aware of. This information may well tie in with recent visits to the doctors or hospital.

Past medical history

This is essential to provide information about the cause of the emergency, and anything that may affect the patient's subsequent treatment. A photocopy of the medical history form is helpful, or written notes that clearly state any conditions the patient is known to have.

Last oral intake

Airway complications are common in patients who become acutely ill. The paramedic crew can receive important information regarding possible problems in maintaining an airway by finding out when the patient last ate. A shocked patient runs a high risk of vomiting, and the likelihood of this happening increases when the stomach is full. The decision of whether the patient should be intubated could rest on the dental team investigating the patient's recent ingestion of food.

Events before the incident

A comprehensive history should include those events that took place leading up to the emergency and the 999 call. If the patient was suffering from a crushing substernal chest pain the paramedics would want to know for how long the patient had the pain. If the patient had an anaphylactic crisis it would be helpful to inform the paramedics of any allergens you suspected.

Step 4 — Informing a Relative

It is always good practice to ensure that dental surgeries have recorded contact details of a person the patient would wish to be contacted in the event of an emergency. If a patient is to be transferred to hospital then this person should be contacted and informed about the nature of the emergency and which hospital the patient has been transferred to — this must be done sensitively and carefully to avoid causing panic. The paramedics will also need to know this information to pass on to the hospital.

Medical History

- Do you know where the patient's medical history is recorded?
- Do you routinely check it before the patient is in the surgery?
- Do the patient's fill a form in themselves? If the answer is yes does somebody go though it with the patient to verify it.
- Do you check if there has been any change in the patients medical history since their last visit?

Chair Position

- Do you know how to quickly change the dental chair position?
- Can you adjust the position from the nurses side of the chair?

Emergency Equipment

- Do you know where the oxygen cylinder is?
- Can you turn the oxygen cylinder on?
- How often do you check how full the oxygen cylinder is?
- How low must the oxygen cylinder be before you replace it?
- How many oxygen cylinders are in your practice, do you know exactly where the other cylinders are in case yours runs out?
- Where are the non-rebreathing masks?
- Can you attach them to the oxygen supply?
- Where are the pocket masks kept
- Can you remove a pocket mask from the box and assemble it?
- Can you attach the pocket mask correctly to the oxygen tubing and what flow rate would you use?
- Where are the bag/valve masks kept?
- Can you assemble a bag, valve mask and correctly attach one to the oxygen supply?
- Where is the emergency portable suction and can you use it?
- Can it be used easily anywhere on the premises?

Training in the Management and Prevention of Medical Emergencies

- Can you open an airway correctly on a simulator?
- Can you correctly use a face mask on a simulator and deliver effective ventilations?
- Can you correctly use a bag, valve mask on a simulator and deliver effective ventilations?
- Can you place a patient in the recovery position?
- Do you know how to deliver an abdominal thrust?
- Can you effectively count a respiration rate?
- Can you take a pulse?
- Can you measure blood pressure?
- Can you measure CRT?
- Can you deliver effective cardiac compressions on a simulator?
- Do you have a defibrillator and can you assemble it?
- Do you have a blanket in the practice?
- Can you measure blood glucose?
- Do you know where the emergency drug kit is kept?
- Do you know what is in the emergency drug kit?
- Can you assemble the drug preparations ready for administration?
- Do you know how to contact the paramedics?
- Do you know what information they will need?
- Do you hold scenario practices within your teams in the surgery?

Useful Sources of Information

Asthma UK: for specific information about asthma.
Website: *www.asthsma.org.uk*

Diabetes UK: for specific information about diabetes.
Website: *www.diabetes.org.uk*

British National Formulary: has a comprehensive guide to drugs and drug interactions and it carries a list of drugs required to be available in dental surgeries. This publication is updated every 6 months.
Website: *www.bnf.org*

Bupa: for health factsheets of specific conditions.
Website: *www.hcd2.bupa.co.uk*

General Dental Council: for information on continuing professional development requirements and standards.
Website: *www.bnf.org*

Mayo Clinic: for descriptions of causes, signs and symptoms of medical conditions, together with information on presentation, management and prognosis.
Website: *www.mayoclinic.com*

Medicines Information Service: can provide advice on drug therapy relating to dentistry.
Website: *www.nyrdtc.nhs.uk*

Medic 8*:* for descriptions of causes, signs and symptoms of medical conditions, together with information on presentation, management and prognosis.
Website: *www.medic8.com*

NHS Direct: for definitions of medical conditions and general information and references.
Website: *www.nhsdirect.nhs.uk*

Patient.co.uk: for descriptions of causes, signs and symptoms of medical conditions, together with information on presentation, management and prognosis.
Website: *www.patient.co.uk*

Resuscitation Council UK: for current and updated guidelines on all aspects of resuscitation.
Website: *www.resus.org.uk*.
For specific information on the Standards expected for dental care professionals you can download the document *Medical Emergencies and Resuscitation — Standards for Clinical Practice and Training for Dental Practitioners and Dental Care professionals in General Dental Practice 2006*, available at: *www.resus.org.uk/pages/MEdental.pdf*

Stroke Association: for specific information about CVAs and TIAs.
Website: *www.stroke.org.uk*

Postgraduate Dental Deaneries

These will have details of medical emergencies courses and BLS training providers in your local areas:

DEANERY	NAME	ADDRESS	WEBSITE
Eastern	Alex Baxter Director of Postgraduate Dental Education	Posgraduate Medical and Dental Education Eastern Deanery Block 3 Ida Darwin Site Fulbourn Cambridge CBI 5EE	www.nhseducationoeo.nhs.uk
Kent/Surrey/Sussex	Stephen Lambert-Humble Dean of Postgraduate Dentistry	The KSS Deanery 7 Bermondsey Street London SEI 2DD	www.kssdeanery.ac.uk

Continued...

Leeds/Yorkshire	Paul Cook Postgraduate Dental Dean	University of Leeds Department for NHS Postgraduate Medical and Dental Education Willow Terrace Road Leeds LS2 9JT	www.yorkshiredeanery.com
London	Elizabeth Jones Dean of Postgraduate Dentistry	Dental Department LPMDE Stewart House 32 Russell Square London WC1B 5DN	www.londondeanery.ac.uk
Mersey	Brian Grieveson Dean of Postgraduate Dental Education and Training	The University of Liverpool Department of Postgraduate Dental Education and Training Fisrt Floor Regatta Place Brunswick Business Park Summers Road Liverpool L3 6BL	www.merseydeanery.ac.uk
North West	Nick Ward Dean of Postgraduate Dentistry	North Westyern Deanery 4th Floor Barlow House Minshull Street Manchester M1 3DZ	www.pgmd.man.ac.uk
Northern	Malcolm Smith Acting Postgraduate Dental Dean	University of Newcastle Postgraduate Institute for Medicine and Dentistry 10–12 Framlington Place Newcastle Upon Tyne NE2 4AB	www.pimd.co.uk
Oxford	Helen Falcon Postgraduate Dental Dean	Oxford University Oxford Postgraduate Medical and Dental Education The Triangle Roosevelt Drive	www.oxdent.ac.uk

Continued...

South West	Alasdair Miller Regional Postgraduate Dental Dean	University of Bristol Dental Postgraduate Department The Chapter House Bristol Dental Hospital Lower Maudlin Street Bristol BS1 2LY	www.swdentalpg.net
South Yorkshire/East Midlands	Chris Franklin Postgraduate Dental Dear	Regional Postgraduate Dental Education Office Don valley House Savile Street East Sheffield S4 7UQ	www.pgdetrent.co.uk
West Midlands	John Frame Postgraduate Dental Dean	University of Birmingham Postgraduate Office Dental School St Chad's Queensway Birmingham B4 6NN	www.pgdentistrybham.ac.uk
Northern Ireland	David Hussey Postgraduate Dental Dean	NIMDTA Beechill House 42 Beechill Road Belfast BT8 7RS	www.nimdta.gov.uk
Scotland	David Felix Associate Dean for Postgraduate Dental Education	NHS Education for Scotland Hanover Buildings 66 Rose Street Edinburgh EH2 2NN	www.news.scot.nhs.uk
Wales	Eric Nash Director of Postgraduate Dental Education	University of Cardiff Dental Postgraduate Depatment Room 130 Dental School Heath park Cardiff CF14 4XY	www.dentpostgradwales.ac.uk

INDEX

A

ABCDE approach 75
Abdominal thrust 11
Adjuncts 16
Adrenaline 71, 87, 133
  epinephrine 60
Adrenal shock 129
Age 90
Airway 76
Airway maintenance 16
Airways 98
Alcohol 38, 90
Allergens 100
Allergies 139
Amphetamines
  cocaine 38
Ampoules. *See also* Injections
Anaesthetics 132
Anaphylaxis 72, 83–88
Angina 72, 89–96, 92
Anticonvulsant medication 110
Anxiety 36
Arm weakness 105
Aspirin 60, 69
Assessment 75–82. *See also* Central
     Nervous System
Asthma 72, 97–102
Asthma UK 143
Atrial fibrillation 80
AVPU scale 40

B

Benzodiazepines 112, 134
  Diazepam
    Midazolam 38
Blood pressure 23

Brachial pulse 28
Breathing 76, 109
Breathlessness 94
British National Formulary 143
Bronchodilators
  salbutamol
    terbutaline 100
Bupa 143

C

Carbohydrate 125
Cardiac arrest 30, 53, 72, 94
Cardiac emergencies
  prevention 95
Cardiac output 25
Cardiovascular accident 103
Cardiovascular system 23–34
Carotid pulse 27
Central nervous system 35
Chair position 141
Chest compressions 48
Chest pain 94, 120
Chills 120
Chlorphenamine 71, 87
Chocolate 126
Choking 11
Circulation 25, 77
Collapse 129–136
Consciousness 39
Convulsions 109
Coronary arteries 91
Coronary heart disease 90
Cortisol 131
Cyanosis 99